COMPLEMENTARY MEDICINE

for nurses, midwives and health visitors

Joanna Trevelyan & Brian Booth

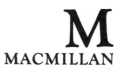

MACMILLAN

First published 1994 by
MACMILLAN PRESS LTD
Houndmills, Basingstoke, Hampshire RG21 2XS
and London
Companies and representatives
throughout the world

Illustrated by Konstantinos Pavlopoulos

ISBN 0–333–59601–3

A catalogue record for this book is available
from the British Library

10   9   8   7   6   5   4   3   2   1
03 02 01 00 99 98 97 96 95 94

Printed in Great Britain by
Antony Rowe Ltd, Chippenham, Wiltshire

Addresses accurate as of February 1994.

Dedication

To Costi and Sue, who have endured so much; and Michael and Jonathan, conceived months after the start of this book, but born before the last page was written.

JT
BB

CONTENTS

FOREWORD

Medicine, along with many other areas of modern life, is under regular scrutiny and is in a constant state of flux and development. On the one hand orthodox medicine continues to develop improved medical and surgical techniques for treating all manner of conditions; on the other, along with the transformation of orthodox medical practice, there has been an increase in interest in complementary therapies among both the general public and health professionals, including nurses.

With the growth of complementary medicine in the UK have come a number of problems, as well as opportunities. While there is increasing evidence of wider interest in complementary medicine among nurses and doctors, there is still a strong undercurrent of scepticism and hostility. A burgeoning number of complementary therapy practitioners and wider public usage of complementary medicine do not, of themselves, provide proof of efficacy and safety. The Research Council for Complementary Medicine has spent over ten years encouraging a research ethos in the field. It is clear that the evidence of rigorous scientific research, whether the results were positive or negative, would be one way of meeting the criticism and doubts so often expressed. *Complementary Medicine for Nurses, Midwives and Health Visitors* rightly places considerable emphasis on the value of research and the need for all involved in complementary medicine to understand its significance in the development of professional standards of practice.

The BMA report *Complementary Medicine: new approaches to good practice*, published in June 1993, called for improved training and education within the complementary medicine. It placed particular importance on the need for research as well as for some form of 'familiarisation on complementary medicine' for medical students. The same should hold true for student nurses and midwives. Orthodox medicine is more open to the positive elements of complementary medicine – the need now is for non-medically qualified practitioners to put their own house in order and look to developing closer links with the health service. The recently launched European Union project on Unconventional Medicine, combined with the freedom granted to general practitioners to 'delegate' to complementary practitioners, highlight the opportunities for collaboration which already exist.

The authors of *Complementary Medicine for Nurses, Midwives and Health Visitors* are to be congratulated on trying to present an overview of the situation as it is today in the UK. The growth of complementary medicine has led to the emergence of a wide range of organisations, and to the newcomer this can be somewhat daunting. How do the public know what is a validated and professional therapy or organisation? Where can the evidence be found to support the claims of practitioners in support of the therapies with which they are involved?

It is clear from the excellent response to the recent series of articles on complementary medicine and nursing in the *Nursing Times* that considerable energy and drive are being given to the practice of complementary therapies by an increased perception of their value in nursing practice. The authors of this book are responding to a real need for information, for research and for wider debate as to the best way forward.

Fourteen different therapies are studied in the book: they are presented in a manner which helps clarify some of the strong and weak points about each therapy, some of the principal organisations associated with it, and a selection of some of the published research that might be of interest. The book provides a simple and readable format for the newcomer to complementary medicine.

There is much work still to be done in assessing the efficacy and safety of complementary medicine. As the changes in the NHS continue, and purchasers are required to determine which services to offer, it is important that the public be prudent in their use of the therapies and discerning in their selection of practitioners. The future of complementary medicine depends, to a large extent, on it remaining just that: 'complementary' to orthodox medicine and not an alternative. Appropriate usage, supported by rigorous research, will lead to improved health care for all.

Complementary Medicine for Nurses, Midwives and Health Visitors is an informative and worthwhile read. It will, I hope, lead to more detailed and in-depth reviews of current trends, scientific research and published reviews in the field of complementary medicine.

Jonathan Monckton
Director, Research Council for Complementary Medicine

ACKNOWLEDGEMENTS

This book would not have been possible without the help and co-operation of a large number of practitioners and researchers. To list all their names would be impossible, but we are grateful to everyone who gave us their time, and the benefits of their experience and knowledge, throughout the course of researching and writing this text.

Special thanks are owed to:
Sylvia Baker; Kathleen Ballard; Sally Billings; Richard Brennan; Wainwright Churchill; Frances Clifford; Brenda Cooke; Dr Ian Drysdale; Tony Hampson; Jonathan Hobbs; Judy Howard; Chris Jarmey; Mary Martin; Dr Tony Metcalfe; Nicky Moss-Phillips; Jackie Pietroni; the Research Council for Complementary Medicine (Jonathan Monckton, Jane Buckle, Andrew Vickers); Jean Sayre-Adams; Enid Segall; Jonathan Stallick; The Tisserand Institute; Midge Whiteleg; Timothy Whittaker; Janine Wood; Valerie Ann Worwood; and Sylvia Wright.

1 COMPLEMENTARY MEDICINE TODAY

What's in a name?

Complementary, alternative, traditional, natural, fringe, unorthodox, quack: the therapies and techniques we discuss in this book have been called many things. Which you select reveals a great deal about your views on the subject.

As recently as the 1950s there was no collective name to speak of, although 'quackery' was a term much on the lips of doctors. Then, in the early 1960s, Brian Inglis and Geoffrey Murray coined the phrase 'fringe medicine' (Inglis 1979), apparently inspired by the Fringe at the Edinburgh Festival. The marginalisation implicit in this description made it unlikely to be popular for long (although the *British Medical Journal* – unsurprisingly – quickly adopted it).

By the 1970s, 'fringe' medicine in the UK had become 'natural' medicine, in tune with the 'back to nature' hippie culture of the early part of that decade. Elsewhere in the world, different terms were being used: 'alternative medicine' in the USA, for example; 'other' medicine, in Italy; and in France, 'non-proven', 'parallel' or 'non-official'. The World Health Organisation (WHO) plumped for 'traditional medicine', which seemed fine for developing countries but was confusing in more developed countries, where 'traditional' often means 'conventional' or 'orthodox'.

The term 'complementary' emerged in the 1980s, first being used in 1981 in a report on the status of unorthodox medicine in the UK by a Swiss-based charity called The Threshold Foundation (Fulder & Munro 1981). By 1985 it had appeared in an article in the *Lancet* (Fulder & Munro 1985) and was in common parlance among those who sought to bring orthodox and unorthodox together. The problem with the word 'complementary' is that it suggests that the therapies concerned can only be used as an adjunct to 'orthodox' medicine. Clearly most therapies can be used as a 'complement' to other forms of medicine, but they are also used as the 'treatment of choice' by many people. There are also therapies that still confound scientists seeking to understand the mechanisms by which they work; these cannot easily be described as 'complementary' to orthodox medicine in terms of their theoretical basis. Examples of such therapies include homoeopathy and acupuncture.

Many practitioners prefer the term 'alternative', which, they say, nicely reflects the place of the therapies in the health care system, denotes their independence from orthodox medicine, and fits in with the 'alternative lifestyles' of which they are often part. Most recently, the British Medical Association has opted for 'non-conventional' (BMA 1993).

For this book, like parents choosing a name for their child, we narrowed our choice down to two: 'complementary' and 'alternative'. We chose 'complementary' because you, our readers, will generally see these therapies as 'complementing' your practice, not as 'alternatives' to it. In making this choice, however, we have not intended to make a value judgement, and we respect the right of others to claim these therapies as alternatives to conventional medicine, rather than as complements.

But what are we referring to when we talk about complementary medicine? Inglis believes complementary medicine can best be defined by the approach it uses. He likens it to that advocated in the mid 19th century by Claude Bernard, that 'Health is best preserved'. According to Inglis (1993), this is achieved 'not by finding ways to eliminate disease agents with the help of drugs, but by looking after the terrain, as he [Bernard] called it, to ensure that our immune systems are in good working order ... against that, the discoveries of the microbe hunters led to the hope that diseases could be wiped out at source by "magic bullets".'

The WHO defines complementary medicine as those forms of medicine that 'usually lie outside the official health sector', but the danger with this definition is that it lumps together an enormous number of wildly different therapies, from the well established to the frankly dubious. More useful, argues West (1992), is a categorisation which divides complementary medicine into two different types, 'those that require a high degree of professional training and skill and those that are at heart variations on first aid, do-it-yourself, and self-care techniques'.

While accepting this division, we have chosen to group the therapies included here according to the use that you, our readers, might make of them:

- those which you might reasonably incorporate within your practice after appropriate training – massage, shiatsu, reflexology, aromatherapy, and Therapeutic Touch;
- those of which you are unlikely to become practitioners (because of the extent of training required), but which offer some scope for personal use in the form of readily available remedies or techniques – nutritional therapies, hypnotherapy, homoeopathy, herbal medicine, and naturopathy; and

- those which you are unlikely to incorporate within your practice in any form (again because of the extent of training required), but about which you should be able to inform your patients: acupuncture, chiropractic, osteopathy, and the Alexander technique.

These groupings are indicated by the shaded bars at the sides of the pages.

The meaning of holism

Another term closely associated with complementary medicine is 'holism', or 'wholism'. *The Concise Oxford Dictionary* (Sykes 1983) defines this as the 'tendency in nature to form wholes that are more than the sum of the parts by ordered grouping'. In relation to health, however, holism refers to an approach to caring for a patient which takes into account social, emotional and spiritual concerns as well as physical and psychological ones.

Invariably complementary therapies are described as holistic, and the fact that they are is often given as evidence of their superiority over conventional medicine. But, as Inglis (1979) points out, 'all this means is that they try to treat the patient, rather than simply the patient's symptoms'. Moreover, not all complementary practitioners are holistic, and many conventional health professionals are.

A look at the past

Unorthodox and orthodox practitioners have been slugging it out in the health arena for many years. Although the sorts of medicine each has practised have changed, one can argue that the two groups have always reflected two different schools of thought: vitalism versus mechanism. Essentially, the vitalists argue that psychological, psychic or spiritual forces are responsible for disease, and that these forces must be invoked if a patient is to recover. The shamanistic and healing traditions are, for example, based on such a premise. The mechanists, on the other hand, seek a physical cause for illness – developing a cold after getting caught in the rain, for example – and will posit a physical treatment to remedy it.

Generally, orthodox medical practitioners have tended to favour the mechanistic view – on the trail of ever more powerful 'magic bullets' to deal with the multiplicity of diseases which affect humankind. Unorthodox, or complementary, practitioners, on the other hand, operate primarily within the vitalist arena. In a sense, orthodox medicine is bound in with rationalism, the scientific revolution and the mind–body split so elegantly argued by Descartes. Its very name – 'orthodox' – describes its place within the establishment, and therefore its access to power. By contrast, complementary medicine represents the medicine of the people, tied in as it is with folklore and tradition, and based on wisdom that was often passed down orally from generation to generation. In the past, its practitioners were the people to whom those too poor to seek out a physician turned for help.

The founding of the College of Physicians of London and the licensing of the apothecaries and surgeons in the early 16th century are convenient starting points for what was to become a division of medicine into orthodox and unorthodox. This division was further strengthened by the Witchcraft Acts of 1542, which worked against folk practitioners. Women healers, including mid-wives, suffered particularly as a result of these Acts.

But complementary medicine did not die in the flames that consumed many of its practitioners. Instead, by the 18th century it was flourishing in the forms of healing, bone-setting and herbalism. By the 19th century, however, the rise of orthodox medicine began in earnest: with the Medical Registration Act of 1858, and with various measures designed either to discredit complementary practitioners, as in the case of mesmerism (see Chapter 9), or to prevent complementary practitioners from posing a threat to doctors, as in the case of homoeopathy (see Chapter 10).

In the first half of the 20th century, orthodox medical control of health care increased, this ascent being supported by the governments of the day. Complementary therapies such as osteopathy failed to win official recognition and, in a sense, the public health service became the 'orthodox health service'. When the National Health Service came into being in 1948, only one of the complementary therapies, homoeopathy, was incorporated within it.

By the 1960s, however, change was in the air. Among other things, the thalidomide disaster shook public confidence in orthodox medicine; the ecological movement emerged; and acupuncture came to the West as China was opened up. Complementary medicine staged a comeback and there were even early attempts during the 1960s to unify the field with the setting up of the British Federation of Practitioners of Natural Therapeutics. In the 1970s, the complementary therapies began the slow process of professionalisation with the setting up of colleges and professional organisations, although standards varied widely.

The past decade has seen this process continue. Organisations such as the Research Council for Complementary Medicine and the Council for Complementary and Alternative Medicine (see 'Resources') emerged as champions of the cause of complementary medicine: seeking respectively to demonstrate the validity and efficacies of the therapies, and to protect therapists' right to practise. In 1983, the Prince of Wales became President of the BMA – their 150th year. He used the opportunity to make his now famous speech attacking technological medicine. The BMA (1986) responded with an 'investigation' of what they referred to as 'alternative medicine'. At best this was a less than even-handed exercise, but, as Mills (1993) points out, it 'acted to unite the groups of complementary professionals in outrage'.

The BMA, in seeking to discredit complementary medicine, was in fact out of step with some of its membership. For example, 1983 also saw the publication of a survey of young doctors (Reilly 1983) which showed that 80 per cent would like to train in a complementary therapy, and that some were already referring patients to complementary therapists.

Since the 1980s there has been an increasing integration of complementary medicine within mainstream health services, as this book attests. Complementary therapists have worked hard to gain recognition, the most notable success being the Osteopaths Act 1993 (see Chapter 15). The challenge of the 1990s is likely to be Europe, as the EU seeks to regulate and unify training standards in complementary medicine across Europe. If complementary medicine emerges triumphant from this potential battle it will have ensured its future, and the continuation of choice in the healthcare services which can only be of benefit to those who use them.

How popular is complementary medicine?

In 1980, The Threshold Foundation commissioned a survey of complementary medicine practitioners (Fulder & Munro 1981). It found that the number of consultations was increasing at the rate of 10–15 per cent per year, and estimated that complementary medicine was growing five times as rapidly as orthodox medicine. A recent investigation by Taylor Nelson Medical (West 1992), a marketing research company, found that 1 per cent of the population of Britain use an acupuncturist, 2 per cent use a homoeopath, and 7 per cent use natural medicines on a self-help basis. Other surveys undertaken since 1986 also suggest that interest in, and use of, complementary therapies is widespread and enthusiastic (see Box 1.1).

This popularity is, among other things, both a product and a reflection of some of the profound changes in health awareness and health care that have occurred during the latter half of the 20th century. The combination of the successes of modern medicine, improved sanitation, better diet and the whole gamut of social improvements enshrined within the welfare state, has led to greatly improved health, longer lives and higher expectations of good health among the vast majority of people in Britain. In general we are also better educated and therefore more willing to examine carefully, and to question, the value of anything that others propose to do to us.

When cracks appeared in the armour of orthodox medicine, therefore – unpleasant side-effects of particular treatment regimes; pharmaceutical disasters such as thalidomide; the apparent inability of modern medicine to treat chronic diseases such as myalgic encephalomyelitis (ME), chronic fatigue syndrome, or repetitive strain injury (RSI); the appearance of diseases like AIDS that so far elude a cure, despite the millions of pounds already invested in the research; the emergence of drug-resistant strains of bacteria and viruses; and the slow disintegration of the NHS as patient numbers soar and resources dwindle – the general public began to seek alternatives in earnest.

This move towards complementary medicine also reflects a change in attitude to health and illness. As Coward (1989) argues,

> people's expectations of health, and their sense of personal involvement in it have changed. So too have beliefs about how much they can exercise conscious 'choice' over health and disease. Even the conception of disease has changed: disease is no longer understood either as the curse of mankind or as a completely arbitrary pheonomenon. Instead disease and well-being are both seen as having direct personal 'meanings'. And through the notion of holism, with its implicit privileging of the mind over the body, the 'meaning' of disease is more often than not located in the individual's state of mind.

Interest in complementary medicine has also been fuelled by an increasing awareness of the environment, and by a resultant desire to promote more 'natural' ways of life. Green politics, said Fritjof Capra and Charlene Spretnak (1984), 'emphasises the interconnectedness and interdependence of all phenomena, as well as the embeddedness of individuals and societies in the cyclical process of nature'. These sentiments have echoed in the world of complementary medicine.

BOX 1.1
USE OF COMPLEMENTARY MEDICINE IN THE UK

The Daily Telegraph **questionnaire**

In 1993, *The Daily Telegraph* received 5486 replies to a questionnaire on 'alternative medicine'. A random sample of 1000 was then analysed at the Open University. About 75 per cent of the respondents were women; 50 per cent were aged between 45 and 64; and about 33 per cent were over 65. As many as 96 per cent said they has used an 'alternative therapy'. When asked why, 52 per cent said it was because orthodox treatment was not helping, and 25 per cent because they were worried about the side-effects of orthodox treatment. Of those responding, 77 per cent found the alternative therapy 'very helpful', 17 per cent 'quite helpful', and 94 per cent said they would use the therapy again. The most-used therapies were homoeopathy, osteopathy, acupuncture, medical herbalism, aromatherapy and chiropractic.

– Doyle, C. 1993. Reaching out for an alternative. *The Daily Telegraph*, 6 April.

MCRU investigation

In 1991, researchers from the Medical Care Research Unit in Sheffield investigating the 'use of non-orthodox and conventional health care in Great Britain' estimated that there were 1909 practitioners actively using one of the study treatments (acupuncture, chiropractic, homoeopathy, medical herbalism, naturopathy, and osteopathy) in the UK in 1987. They concluded that: 'Practitioners' own estimates of their normal workload suggested that this group of "non-orthodox" practitioners undertook four million consultations in 1987, roughly one for every 55 patient consultations with a general practitioner in the NHS'. Some 63 per cent were women; 64 per cent of all patients surveyed reported having received orthodox treatment for their main problem from the GP or a hospital specialist before going to the non-orthodox practitioner; 24 per cent reported also being in receipt of concurrent conventional treatment.

– Thomas, K. J., J. Carr, L. Westlake & B. T. Williams 1991. Use of non-orthodox and conventional health care in Great Britain. *British Medical Journal* 302: 207–10.

Consumers' Association survey

In 1986 the Consumers' Association reported that of 28 000 *Which?* members asked, about one in seven said they had used some form of alternative or complementary medicine during the previous twelve months. A more detailed survey was also sent to a smaller sample randomly selected from members who had used alternative or complementary therapies. Of the 1942 who responded, 31 per cent said they had been cured, and 51 per cent that the condition for which they had sought help had improved. Only 14 per cent said the treatment was ineffective, and 1 per cent that their problem had got worse after the treatment. Some 74 per cent said they would 'definitely use this form of medicine again'. The most common types of therapies consulted were: osteopathy (42 per cent), homoeopathy (28 per cent), acupuncture (23 per cent), chiropractic (22 per cent), and herbalism (11 per cent). When asked if they had tried conventional medicine for their problem, 81 per cent said they had been to their GP, but 81 per cent also said they had been dissatisfied because they had not been cured, only got temporary relief, or could not be treated.

– Consumers' Association 1986. Magic or medicine? Which? (October), 443–7.

Who's regulating whom in complementary medicine?

Although the past thirty years have seen many attempts, the sad fact is that, as a group, the complementary therapies have so far failed to 'put their house in order' to the satisfaction of their critics.

Good research into the efficacy of complementary therapies is hard to come by; training standards vary enormously across the therapies, and even within particular therapies; not every therapy has an enforceable regulatory mechanism; and in the UK anyone – with or without training – can set up as a complementary therapist. Attempts to bring therapies together under one roof have led to in-fighting, and to date there is still no overall representative body.

To be fair, the sheer diversity of therapies that practise under the complementary banner, and the widely differing training require-ments of individual therapies, do make this difficult. As Goodliffe (1990) puts it, 'How can a single organisation develop coherent minimum standards for practices as varied as osteopathy (currently requiring a four-year full-time training) and reflexology (which might be studies over a number of weekends)?'

And it is not hard to understand why acupuncturists, for example, whose discipline has a sound research base and well-regulated train-ing standards, would not want to be lumped together with, say, crystal healing, which remains a largely untested therapy. This goes a long way towards explaining why some 'umbrella organisations' attract one sort of membership, others a quite different one.

The Council for Complementary and Alternative Medicine (CCAM – see 'Resources'), for example, was set up in 1985 to represent what might be called the 'major' therapies, such as acupuncture, herbal-ism, homoeopathy, naturopathy and osteopathy. Its formation was a response to the Government's advice that it wanted to deal with a unified representation of complementary medicine. However, CCAM now recognises that an umbrella organisation is not a long-term solution. The Government too has changed its mind. According to Baroness Hooper (1990), it now believes 'very firmly that it must be for each therapy group to determine its own future development'.

'Umbrella organisations' which are still trying to bring therapies together, however, include the Institute for Complementary Medicine (ICM) and the relatively new group, the British Complementary Medicine Association (BCMA – see 'Resources'). Each has a rather eclectic membership, including anything from polarity therapy, through massage, to iridology. In the main they both represent the less well-established, less-regulated therapies. Both organisations seek to improve standards and are looking at the introduction of National Vocational Qualifications, which would give a basic standard for many of the smaller untested therapies. This development can only be viewed as a 'good thing'.

Before leaving the subject of regulation, it is worth mentioning another problem. With its enormous popularity among the general public there is obviously a lot of money to be made from complementary medicine, and this has attracted all manner of people to the party. At the fringes of complementary medicine are some highly dubious therapies set up by people with no ostensible qualifications. There are also, it seems, an awful lot of manufacturers peddling the modern equivalents of magical charms and religious relics to the more gullible sections of the population. These activities bring into disrepute all complementary therapies, and provide ammunition for critics.

Complementary medicine and the health service

The status and use of complementary medicine in the health service has changed a great deal since the early 1980s, when the best that could be said was that 80 per cent of young GPs were interested in training in a complementary therapy (Reilly 1983), and that a small band of health professionals had got together to form the British Holistic Medical Association to promote holistic care (see 'Resources') among doctors, nurses and other paramedics.

According to the Department of Health (DoH), GPs in England employed, in 1993, the equivalent of 169 'whole-time' complementary therapists. Since such therapists would be likely only to be employed for a few sessions a week at most, this means that up to 1700 GPs could be employing a therapist for a morning or afternoon a week.

A report by the National Association of Health Authorities and Trusts (NAHAT), published in April 1993, has also revealed that the NHS as a whole is prepared to purchase complementary therapies such as acupuncture, osteopathy, homoeopathy and chiropractic for patients, and that approximately £1 million is already being spent annually on these services.

This national survey by NAHAT aimed to find out about purchasers' attitudes towards the availability of complementary therapies in the NHS, and their current and future approaches to purchasing complementary therapies. Questionnaires were sent to all 191 district health authorities (DHAs), all 98 family health services authorities (FHSAs) and a sample of GP fundholders (GPFHs). Response rates of 57 per cent for DHAs, 75 per cent for FHSAs and 43 per cent for GPFHs were achieved.

More than 70 per cent of FHSAs and GPFHs and 65 per cent of DHAs responding to the survey were in favour of some or all of these services being freely available at the point of contact. Of the districts, 92 were funding therapies via contracts or as extra-contractual referrals. Many FHSAs (55) had been approached for the approval of health-promotion clinics involving complementary therapies; 44 of these had given their approval.

However, the report warned that 'Funding complementary therapies is generally not considered a high priority in a system of finite resources in which there are already difficulties in funding therapies of proven effectiveness and achieving an appropriate balance of basic practice staff in primary care'. It also concluded that 'A critical review of all available evidence on the effectiveness of complementary therapies needs to be undertaken'; recommended an investigation of the cost benefits of complementary medicine; and emphasised the importance of developing standards for training.

An important contributing factor in this change of culture within the health service was the announcement by Stephen Dorrell in 1991, when he was a junior minister at the DoH, that GPs could employ complementary therapists in their practices provided that they themselves remained responsible for the patients' care and felt that the complementary therapy being offered would benefit their patients.

The Labour party, too, has jumped on the bandwagon. Before the general election in 1992, it said that, under a Labour administration, certain complementary disciplines would have a place in the NHS of the future. In June 1993 it produced a consultation document entitled *Complementary Medicine: new approaches to good practice*, which called for selected therapies to be brought within the NHS, free at the point of service.

Interestingly, a survey by *The Daily Telegraph* (see Box 1.1 for more details) found that, of readers who responded to their questionnaire, only 33 per cent were aware that GPs could 'delegate' patients to be treated by a complementary therapist; 18 per cent that budget-holding GPs can purchase complementary therapy treatment, and 11 per cent that non-budget-holding GPs can apply to their FHSA to employ or fund complementary therapists. About 67 per cent of respondents said that they would now consider asking their GP for a complementary therapy under the NHS. Replies from GPs found that 66 per cent thought that some therapies should be available on the NHS: 26 per cent thought that all therapies should be available, and 28 per cent that therapists should be medically qualified (Doyle 1993).

Nurses, too, have become enthusiastic proponents of complementary therapies (see Chapter 2 for details); the Royal College of Nursing now has a special-interest group in complementary medicine which boasts more than two thousand members, and has collaborated with complementary therapists to produce a massage course for nurses. Study days and courses on complementary medicine for nurses are being run all over the UK by a variety of organisations, and small research studies by nurses are increasingly being reported in the nursing press. Indeed, Labour's consultative document calls for more training for nurses who would, says the report, 'have a large role in the delivery of other complementary therapies'.

In response to an increasing use of complementary therapies by health professionals, some health authorities are developing operational policies for the use of complementary therapies by health-authority staff. For example, Bath District Health Authority has formulated a local policy for the use of complementary therapies by nurses (Armstrong & Waldron 1991). This policy clarifies which nurses would be competent to practise complementary therapies and lays down guidelines on patient consent, consultation with medical colleagues, authorisation by nurse managers, and documentation in patient care plans.

Another recent development has been co-operative projects between the health service and complementary therapists or organisations. For example, a visit in 1988 by oncologists from Hammersmith Hospital in London to the Bristol Cancer Help Centre (which offers alternative cancer treatment) resulted in a joint development programme 'in which the Bristol expertise was integrated with that of an academic oncology unit' (Burke & Sikora 1992). A supportive care programme was developed at Hammersmith, which aims 'to treat and care for patients and their families in terms of physical, social, emotional and spiritual needs'. This includes offering patients a variety of complementary therapies and self-help techniques – all of which are part of an ongoing evaluation.

Even the BMA, not known for its support of complementary therapies, has had a change of heart. In 1986 it published a report by a working party set up 'to consider the feasibility and possible methods of assessing the value of alternative therapies, whether used alone or to complement other treatments, and to report on the evidence received to the Board of Science and Education'. It concluded that there might be more to some alternative therapies than simply a placebo effect, but only a strong dose of double-blind trials would sort the matter out once and for all. In the meantime the working party recommended (BMA 1986) that if a patient decides to seek the 'non-specific help offered by, for example, an aromatherapist', doctors should ensure that the patient is 'helped to understand that consultation with the practitioners of some alternative therapies may be attended by the risk of great harm'.

In June 1993 the BMA published the findings of a new investigation. The brief this time was 'to set up a working party to consider the practice and use of complementary medicine since 1985 throughout the UK and the European Economic Community, and its implications following the completion of the single market after 1992'. Its conclusions and tone are rather different from the 1986 report, which dismissed alternative medicine as a 'passing fashion'. They include the following recommendations:

- 'priority should be given to research in acupuncture, chiropractic, herbalism, homoeopathy, and osteopathy as the therapies most commonly used in this country';
- 'The Council of Europe co-operation in Science and Technology (COST) project on non-conventional therapies [should] be approved by the UK Government';
- 'Accredited postgraduate sessions [should] be set up to inform clinicians on the techniques used by different therapists and the possible benefits for patients ... consideration should be given to the inclusion of a familiarisation course on non-conventional therapies within the medical undergraduate curriculum'.

And what of the future? According to West (1992), there are three possible scenarios:

In one, we continue much as we are. The economy survives; material well-being is maintained; and the health services are extended, modified, and improved to cope with an increasing population that is weighted towards old age. In a second, disaster strikes, and we are in a life-boat economy. Alternative medicine takes up a 'barefoot doctor' role in the struggle to provide any kind of health care. In the third, society is transformed. People change from being 'outer-directed', looking for the achievement of material goals, to becoming self-explorers, seeing inner growth as the way forward. Alternative medicine takes its place as a resource for self-care, leading to health, well-being and personal development.

It remains to be seen which of these scenarios, if any, becomes a reality.

Complementary medicine and the European Union

Complementary therapies, vitamins, minerals, and herbal and homoeopathic remedies have all, at some point, come under the scrutiny of the European Commission (Goodliffe 1990; Trevelyan 1990). The situation is confusing as member states differ greatly in what therapies can be practised within their countries and which remedies can legally be sold to their populations. In France and Belgium, for example, it is illegal to practise complementary therapies unless you are a doctor; in Italy traditional herbal remedies are widely used and increasingly popular; and in Denmark complementary therapists practise in much the same way as in the UK.

Various directives have been formulated, or are in the process of being formulated, including a homoeopathic directive which states that 'patients should be allowed access to the medicinal products of their choice' (see Chapter 10).

So far, the EU has been slow to put out specific training directives – not least because of the wildly different situations that exist in member states. Already in existence is a directive which lays down the EU's system for the recognition of higher-education diplomas awarded on completion of professional education and training of at least three years' duration (Lewith & Aldridge 1991). It is clear that some complementary therapies will be able to satisfy the terms of this directive: for example two schools of osteopathy already offer degree courses to students. Certainly many other therapies in the UK are also working towards ensuring that their training programmes meet current EU legislation. Aromatherapists and massage therapists, among others, are actively investigating the introduction of National Vocational Qualifications to their therapies; and other therapies may well begin to offer degree courses in the near future.

Fears in this country that Eurocrats in Brussels would prevent complementary therapists from practising unless they were medically qualified must now be receding. One can only hope they will not be replaced by a fear that the therapies will fail to regulate themselves in a way that protects the public from unscrupulous practitioners.

Resources

Who's who in complementary medicine

Research Council for Complementary Medicine (RCCM)
60 Great Ormond Street, London WC1N 3JF.

The Council, was founded in 1983 to increase medical and practitioner awareness of the need for research into complementary medicine. Its aims are:

- the promotion of scientific research into complementary medicine;
- the dissemination of research results;
- improved collaboration between orthodox and complementary practitioners;
- closer international links among researchers and governments.

The RCCM has charitable status and has retained its neutrality, neither promoting nor condemning, but rather investigating the efficacy of, the different therapies. As a result it has good working relationships within the Medical Research Council, the British Medical Association, the Medicines Control Agency, and the World Health Organisation. The RCCM also has an information service based on an extensive research database.

Council for Complementary and Alternative Medicine (CCAM)
179 Gloucester Place, London NW1 6DX.

The Council was launched in 1985 to provide a forum for communication and co-operation between professional bodies representing acupuncture, herbal medicine, homoeopathy and osteopathy. The objects of the Council include the following:

- to establish and maintain a forum for determining standards of education, training, qualification, ethics and discipline for practitioners of complementary and alternative medicine for the protection and benefit of the public;
- to seek statutory registration for all or any of the member bodies of the Council who may be desirous of such registration as and when appropriate;
- to preserve freedom of choice for members of the public to select their means of health care.

Institute for Complementary Medicine (ICM)
PO Box 194, London SE16 1QZ.

The Institute was set up in 1982 'to ensure that high standards of practice and training in natural health care were available to the public'. Some 230 organisations and training schools are affiliated to the ICM, and a further 200 are associated.

The Institute also runs the British Register of Complementary Practitioners and the British Council of Complementary Medicine.

The ICM has a library and information service; runs introductory courses for nurses and doctors 'to facilitate their work with complementary therapy practitioners'; and is 'linked to universities and other educational organisations with a view to achieving recognition of complementary medical training courses – in particular, the development of National Vocational Qualifications (NVQs) for complementary therapies.

The ICM has worked with the Royal College of Nursing to develop courses for nurses wishing to train in complementary therapies.

British Holistic Medical Association (BHMA)
179 Gloucester Place, London NW1 6DX.

The BHMA was set up in 1983 for 'doctors, para-medical professionals and complementary practitioners who are dedicated to the holistic approach to health care'. The aims of the BHMA are:

- educating doctors and other health-care professionals in the principles and practise of holistic medicine;
- encouraging research studies and the publication of work carried out in the field of holistic medicine;
- bringing together holistic health-care practitioners for mutual support and further personal and professional development.

British Complementary Medicine Association (BCMA)
St Charles Hospital, Exmoor Street, London W10 6DZ.

The BCMA was launched in 1992 as 'the only democratic umbrella organisation established to represent the interests of the natural therapies'. The BCMA claims a membership of more than forty organisations in thirty therapies. The Association has a register of more than twenty thousand practitioners available to the general public, and a code of conduct by which members must abide.

Natural Medicines Society (NMS)
Edith Lewis House, Ilkeston, Derbyshire DE7 8EJ.

The Natural Medicines Society was set up in 1985 'to protect and develop natural and holistic medicine'. Its activities include sponsoring research, training and education, with the aim of promoting 'awareness and understanding of natural medicines and their proper contribution to health'. The Society is also actively involved as an advocate for natural medicines in debates in the UK and Europe.

Centre for Complementary Health Studies
University of Exeter, Streatham Court, Rennes Drive, Exeter EX4
4PU.

The Centre is both a research and a teaching unit, and now has a chair in complementary medicine. The Centre offers a two-year Bachelor of Philosophy course to doctors, nurses and complementary practitioners, and higher degrees can also be taken.

References

- Armstrong, F. & R. Waldron 1991. A complementary strategy. *Nursing Times* **87**(11): 34–5.
- BMA 1986. *Alternative Therapy. Report of the Board of Education*. London: British Medical Association.
- BMA 1993. *Complementary Medicine: new approaches to good practice*. Oxford: Oxford University Press.
- Burke, C. & K. Sikora 1992. Cancer – the dual approach. *Nursing Times* **88**(38): 62–6.
- Capra, F. & C. Spretnak 1984. *Green Politics*. New York: E. P. Dutton.
- Coward, R. 1989. *The Whole Truth: the myth of alternative medicine*. London: Faber & Faber.
- Doyle, C. 1993. Reaching out for an alternative. *The Daily Telegraph*, 6 April.
- Fulder, S. J. & R. Munro 1981. *The Status of Complementary Medicine in the United Kingdom*. London: The Threshold Foundation.
- Fulder, S. J. & R. Munro 1985. Complementary medicine in the United Kingdom: patients, practitioners and consultations. *Lancet* **2**: 542–5.
- Goodliffe, H. 1990. Therapies under threat. *Nursing Times* **86**(26): 48–9.
- Hooper, Baroness 1990. Medicine: complementary and conventional treatments. *Hansard* (9 May), **518**: 82. London: HMSO.
- Inglis, B. 1979. *Natural Medicine*. Glasgow: Fontana.
- Inglis, B. 1993. Will alternative ever become mainstream? *The Daily Telegraph*, 5 January.
- Lewith, G. & D. Aldridge 1991. *Complementary Medicine and the European Community*. Saffron Walden: C. W. Daniel.
- Mills, S. 1993. The development of the complementary medical professions. *Complementary Therapies in Medicine* **1**(1): 24–9.
- NAHAT 1993. *Complementary Therapies in the NHS* (Research Paper No. 10). London: National Association of Health Authorities and Trusts.
- Reilly, D. T. 1983. Young doctors' views on alternative medicine. *British Medical Journal* **287**: 337–9.
- Sykes, J. B. (ed.) 1983. *The Concise Oxford Dictionary*. Oxford: Oxford University Press.
- Trevelyan, J. 1990. Unfairly condemned? *Nursing Times* **86**(26): 50–1.
- West, R. 1992. Alternative medicine: prospects and speculations. In Saks, M. (ed.): *Alternative Medicine in Britain*. Oxford: Clarendon Press.

2 NURSING AND COMPLEMENTARY MEDICINE

Chapter 1 looks at the explosion of interest in complementary therapies among the general public; in this chapter, we concentrate on one small part of the population – nurses, midwives and health visitors.

If any nurse researcher is looking for a subject for his or her doctoral thesis, the development of complementary therapies in nursing would make a fascinating subject. Just a few years ago, references in the nursing press to such therapies were few and far between, and the same handful of names kept cropping up again and again. The quality of published material was variable, but it would not be unfair to say that the majority of it would probably stand little chance of getting into a journal today. What *would* be unfair would be to suggest that there was some kind of fault with the authors, for that is not the case: Hippocrates, were he to be resurrected, might find it difficult to get a paper accepted by the *British Medical Journal* or *Lancet*, if sent anonymously; and as nursing and complementary medicine, both singly and in conjunction, have changed beyond recognition, together with their knowledge bases, the most perspicacious writers of the mid-1980s and earlier likewise now seem almost primitive in their lack of sophistication.

Chapter 1 records how increasing numbers of people have turned away from blind acceptance of medical omniscience – whether this is because of increasing health awareness, a dawning realisation that the medical colossus may have feet of clay, or a general 'flight from science' is immaterial. The public now demand more from health-care providers than has ever been expected before, and nurses, as members of the public who are simultaneously part of the health-care establishment – albeit members seeking autonomy within that establishment – cannot help but be affected.

A time of changes

Nursing has changed dramatically over the past fifteen years. Hospital turnover has increased as patients stay for shorter periods, and are discharged in a much less independent state than ever before – one has only to think about patients undergoing abdominal surgery, whose stay is now counted in days, rather than weeks – and this, in turn, has effects on community nursing. Nurses are treating more patients, with higher dependency levels, than ever before, which more than cancels out any increase in numbers of staff that may have been gained.

This should mean that patients are being cared for more intensively, but that is not how many practitioners perceive the reality, believing that, on the contrary, there has been a decrease in the amount of 'hands on' care delivered. Some nurses might say that this is because of increased time spent in completing paperwork; others would say that the real reason is the increasing delegation of 'basic nursing care' to unqualified staff. Whatever the reason, many nurses believe that they have lost a large degree of patient contact in recent years.

This loss of contact, both physical and social, is a serious problem for many members of the profession, as direct patient care – the application of a range of skills, none of which can be learned from a book, in order to improve someone's quality of life – was their sole reason for taking up nursing in the first place. Yet it has been systematically devalued: delivering 'basic nursing care' is a highly-skilled job, but suggestions that it can be left to unqualified members of staff, be they students, auxiliaries or health-care assistants, have led to the term becoming synonymous with 'unskilled practice'. Thus we hear comments such as this: 'We send our common foundation plan students onto elderly care for their first ward experience, because it's good basic care' – which begs the question, what is advanced care?

Clinical grading, which was supposed to reward nurses for 'staying at the bedside', has not had that effect in many areas; to get a G grade, for example, a hospital nurse might have to become a ward manager, exchanging direct caring for supervision and delegation, with a sizable proportion of his or her time devoted to clerical and administrative work.

At the same time, nursing has moved ever closer to achieving autonomy in practice. A major landmark was the publication in 1992 of the UKCC document, *The Scope of Professional Practice*, which took away nurses' need to produce a piece of paper certifying competence every time they wanted to carry out a procedure which someone had designated an 'extended role'. Now it is up to individual nurses to say whether or not they are competent to undertake any task; but if any problems should arise, the onus is on the individual to demonstrate competence.

As nursing is supposed to be a research-based profession, any such demonstration might hinge on the practitioner being able to show 'knowledge of research or evaluation which has demonstrated effective strategies for recognizing and meeting the needs of dependent people and their carers' (Johns 1992). If members of the public are expressing an interest in complementary therapies, has any nurse the right to withhold such therapies from them, without thoroughly researching their therapeutic value first?

Let us look at these two points in turn.

Complementary therapies as autonomous practice

Consider these elements of the complementary therapies which a nurse might reasonably practise in the clinical setting:

- the nurse needs to have undergone some form of recognised training in the therapy, and to have been awarded proof of having successfully completed the course;
- a stated amount of time has to be set aside for treatment, during which other procedures must take a lower priority;
- there has to be some degree of privacy, with little chance of interruption, as the patient and nurse need to communicate freely;
- the delivery is, literally, 'hands on'.

So: we have an autonomous practitioner, delivering care on a one-to-one basis, without rushing or cutting corners, and all within the framework of the *Code of Professional Conduct* – provided that the training is a 'recognised' one (something which is not quite that simple, as later chapters show). Add to that the prestige which may come with having an identified skill; the right practitioners may earn to call themselves 'clinical specialists' (or at least think of themselves in that way – some practitioners using complementary therapies in their wards have apparently set up sophisticated referral systems for colleagues who want them to see patients); and the personal and professional satisfaction that comes from knowing that one is really giving holistic care (rather than just talking about it) – is it any wonder that there has been an upsurge in interest?

Validation of practice

Chapter 17 deals with problems of research into complementary therapies, but it is worth spending just a little time on it here.

In a society which is perceived as becoming increasingly litigious, nurses seem to be more aware than ever about possible legal repercussions from their actions; the extended debate over the use of Eusol in wound management is just one example. Research-based practice offers at least a partial defence; but the 'theory-practice gap' remains.

Because the number of publications by nurse theoreticians is, proportionately, much higher than the number by clinical nurses, it seems to have become accepted that the theory-practice gap is all the practitioners' fault – an amazing reversal of reality, for if a theoretician cannot get his or her theories accepted into practice then, by definition, those theories must be incomplete, and must merit a return visit to the drawing board. The use of complementary therapies, though, is a special case.

Unlike nursing, the people who are seen as professional leaders in complementary medicine tend to be practitioners first and foremost: if they did not treat patients or clients on a regular basis, they would soon lose their pre-eminence. This has its drawbacks, though, as the critical evaluation of any practice benefits from an outside view from time to time. The preparation of this book involved talking to a large number of practitioners of different therapies, and in the ones dealt with in the first chapters in particular, many of those practitioners seemed unable to understand the need for some degree of objective evaluation of their work. 'Of course it's effective – ask any one of my patients' was a typical response, made all the more arresting for the obvious sincerity with which it was delivered. When we suggested to nurses who felt that way that they must have experience of patients who believed their consultant was doing wonders for them, even when it was obvious to everyone else that their condition was static or even deteriorating, this suggestion met with affirmative responses – and yet these was a total failure to see that the same principle might apply to their use of complementary therapies.

According to establishments offering training in complementary therapies, increasing numbers of nurses are making enquiries about courses, and following them through. If this is true – and judging by the volume of papers submitted for publication to nursing journals, it seems to be more than just an attempt to stimulate interest – then the ranks of the therapists are being swollen with professionals who know the value, and the necessity, of validated practice. The constantly improving quality of published material shows that there has been some effect, but it may be that some nurses have been swept away with enthusiasm, forgetting this fundamental tenet.

Resource implications

In a health service into which an 'internal market' has been introduced, and in which almost everything is being fitted with a price tag, there must be financial implications attached to the use of complementary therapies.

The NAHAT report of 1993 showed that the NHS has responded, albeit cautiously, to the possibility of 'buying in' complementary therapies. As some later chapters show, there are several therapeutic techniques whose value seems to be proven, even when the underlying theory remains open to question, and these seem to be the ones that have started a slow process of integration into mainstream medical care. If more and more nurses are expressing an interest in training in these therapies, then it can only be a matter of time before certain questions start being asked, such as these: Is it worthwhile for a district health authority, a trust hospital, a family health service authority or a fund-holding GP practice to pay for nurses to undertake training in a particular therapy that may be in demand? Would it be cheaper than buying the services of an outside therapist? (If it were not, then some nurses might question whether it was worth spending time and money on courses for themselves.)

This raises a second set of questions. If nurses are to be sent on such courses, will they be given any tangible reward for their increased skill and the responsibility that goes with its practice? After all, taking one of the national board courses, or even a second registration, entitles no one automatically to upgrading, or extra pay, with the possible exception of community nursing qualifications. Is there any guarantee that the best course, as opposed to the cheapest, will be offered? And if the practice of these therapies is restricted to nurses, might patients be being deprived of their right to the best available treatment, which could come from someone specialising in a given therapy rather than fitting it in among a number of other duties?

(There is another side to this case: imagine that some relatively easily-learned techniques were found to have some benefits for patients, and health-care assistants were sent off on one-day courses to master them, while trained nurses were told: 'We don't pay you your E grade' – or D, or F, or whatever – 'just so you can rub people's backs'.)

None of these questions can be answered definitively, of course – but that does not mean that they should not be asked.

BOX 2.1

ARE COMPLEMENTARY THERAPIES INCOMPATIBLE WITH RELIGIOUS BELIEF?

An article published in the nursing press in 1992 provoked a storm of response: In 'Alternative roads to hell?' (Gennis 1992), a nurse teacher argued that 'any healing that comes from sources that are opposed to God's will eventually leads to the destruction of the soul and the spirit in Hell'. She went on to quote various sources, who said that involvement in complementary therapies could lead to 'occult involvement', and that some are 'based on religion that is anti-Christian and anti-Jewish'.

The thrust of her argument was that as the *UKCC Code of Professional Conduct* states that practitioners must respect the spiritual beliefs of patients and clients, the use of therapies based on religious practices (specifically, Eastern ones), without explanation of their origins, could be a transgression of the Code.

This raises a number of further questions – should doctors, for example, warn their patients that the Hippocratic oath, under which they practise, derives from a non-Judaeo-Christian source? – but the whole area needs to be addressed, as there will undoubtedly be patients and clients who may feel the same way as the author quoted above.

In a discussion of Therapeutic Touch (see Chapter 7), one nurse noted that a possible solution has been offered by more than one Christian writer: in addition to 'God-given' and 'demonic' power, there is a 'natural' healing power, whose use carries no spiritual connotations (Turton 1988).

In summary, there are many difficult areas in the introduction of complementary therapies into clinical areas, but there are also many exciting possibilities.

If the benefits of such therapies are real, then nursing has an opportunity to take the lead in a major advance in patient care, and to consolidate the gains made by individual efforts to make practice more holistic. The opportunities for research are there, waiting to be taken up by clinical practitioners: useful therapies can be identified and developed, and less useful ones can be dropped from practice. 'Intuitive' nursing (Wondrak 1992), which so many people fear is being lost, might be reclaimed and even developed.

The only note of caution is this: the use of many therapies has been held back by nurses who were worried that disasters could ensue from the over-enthusiastic application of novel treatment techniques. Now the tide is turning, there is a real danger that they could be proved right, with some nurses apparently believing that they can learn all there is to know about a given therapy in a half-day study session.

In a far-sighted move, Bath District Health Authority has produced a local policy on the use of such therapies by nurses, which lays down four criteria for practice: consent (by the patient); consultation (with medical staff); authorisation (agreed between nurse and nurse manager); and documentation (in the patient's notes). This initiative does much to protect both patient and practitioner, and it is to be hoped that other authorities will follow suit (Armstrong & Waldron 1991).

In the meantime, if a nurse wants to use a complementary therapy, and has the patient's or client's permission, he or she should be asked questions in the following areas, before taking it further:

- Details of training received – is this training adequate?
- Diagnosis – what is the therapy being given for?
- Details of intended action, including a written plan, which could go into the nursing notes.
- Time – how long will treatment take, and is the nurse intending to use ward time, or her own?
- Will the patient's or the client's family co-operate?
- Would a professional therapist be better?

After the uncertainty and demoralisation that have dogged nursing in recent years, it is a pleasant change to see something positive on the horizon; it is up to the profession, individually and collectively, to see that this used wisely and well.

BOX 2.2
RCN SPECIAL-INTEREST GROUP FOR COMPLEMENTARY THERAPIES

The RCN's special-interest group in complementary therapies, which now has around two thousand members, asked its steering committee in 1992 to look at therapies which nurses might realistically be able to use.

The committee reported that 'potentially acceptable therapies', providing nurses were appropriately trained, could be divided up into several groups (Stevensen 1992):

- 'Complete systems of healing' included acupuncture, shiatsu, and other therapies with roots in traditional Chinese medicine; osteopathy; chiropractic; homoeopathy; herbal medicine; Bach flower remedies; gem remedies; Australian bush-flower remedies; and reflexology.
- 'Therapeutic modalities' included different types of massage; Therapeutic Touch; spiritual healing; the Alexander technique; hydrotherapy; and aromatherapy (not oral administration).
- Other groups were 'diagnostic methods'; 'self-help'; 'administrative'; 'tactile'; and 'energetic'.

The full list, it should be noted, includes therapies that take several years' full-time study before a practitioner can say he or she is 'appropriately trained', and others that can be learnt in a very short period. It demonstrates, neatly, the difficulty of naming specific therapies that might be used by nurses.

Further reading

– British Medical Association 1993. *Complementary Medicine: new approaches to good practice*. Oxford: Oxford University Press.

- Buckman, R. & K. Sabbagh 1993. *Magic or Medicine? An investigation into healing*. London: Macmillan.
- Grant, B. 1993. *Alternative Health: A–Z of natural healthcare*. London: Optima.
- Inglis, B. 1979. *Natural Medicine*. London: Collins.
- Olsen, K. 1991. *The Encyclopaedia of Alternative Health Care*. London: Piatkus.
- Rankin-Box, D. (ed.) 1988. *Complementary Health Therapies: a guide for nurses and the caring professions*. London: Chapman & Hall.

References

- Armstrong, F. & R. Waldron 1991. A complementary strategy. *Nursing Times* **87**(11): 34–5.
- Gennis, F. 1992. Alternative roads to hell? *Nursing Standard* **6**(44): 42–3.
- Johns, C. 1992. Developing clinical standards. In Robinson, K., & B. Vaughan (eds): *Knowledge for Nursing Practice*. Oxford: Butterworth-Heinemann.
- NAHAT 1993. *Complementary Therapies in the NHS* (Research Paper No. 10). London: National Association of Health Authorities and Trusts.
- Stevensen, C. 1992. Appropriate therapies for nurses to practice. *Nursing Standard* **6**(5): 51–2.
- Turton, P. 1988. Healing: Therapeutic Touch. In Rankin-Box, D. (ed.): *Complementary Health Therapies: a guide for nurses and the caring professions*. London: Chapman & Hall.
- Wondrak, R. 1992. Intuitive actions. *Nursing Times* **88**(33): 41.

3 MASSAGE

Historical background

Touch is one of the earliest senses we develop, and we have put its healing properties to good use. If a part of our body aches, the natural reaction is to rub it gently in the hope that this will relieve the pain and tension. From such small beginnings, therapies such as massage, shiatsu, Therapeutic Touch and reflexology have developed.

Nobody knows when we started using massage as a form of therapy, but the Chinese certainly appear to have been using it as far back as 3000 BC. Massage is mentioned in the *Nei Jing*, a collection of books on Chinese medicine attributed to the Yellow Emperor Huang-Ti (first written around 400 BC). In India, references to massage are to be found in the *Ayur Veda* (written in about 1800 BC); and Egyptian, Japanese and Persian medical texts document massage as being of value in the cure and relief of many conditions.

The first written records of massage in the West date back to ancient Greece. Hippocrates, for example – who called massage *anatripsis* – wrote about its value in, among other things, improving muscle tone and relieving muscular tension. He believed all physicians should be trained in massage. In *The Odyssey*, Homer describes how soldiers were given a massage with oils after battle. Plato and Socrates also write of the restorative powers of massage.

Celsus, the Roman physician, is known to have recommended massage for convalescents, for those who suffered chronic headaches, and for the paralysed. Pliny and Cicero, too, were enthusiastic about the benefits of massage. Pliny, who suffered from asthma, regularly had a massage to help relieve the symptoms.

Another famous Greek physician, Galen, who practised in the 2nd century AD, recommended massage to the gladiators of Pergamum before and after exercise – something we now know reduces the risk of sports injuries by warming and loosening up the muscles.

By the Middle Ages, however, massage had decreased in popularity – a casualty, in part, of the increased importance given by the Church and the medical practitioners of the day to spiritual, rather than physical, well-being.

During the Renaissance, massage returned to favour. For example, Ambroise Paré (1517–90), physician to four French kings, is known to have used massage; so is the Italian doctor Mercurialis (1530–1606), who wrote about the value of massage and gymnastics. In the 19th century, a Swedish doctor called Per Hendrik Ling (1776–1839) developed 'the Swedish Movement Treatment' (a scientific system of massage) after visiting China. 'Swedish massage' became popular among physicians until high-technology medicine claimed their attention.

More recently, complementary therapies have enjoyed another renaissance, and massage is again a popular form of therapy in the UK. Massage has also reappeared as a therapeutic option within the health service. For example, in the 1970s Peter Nixon, a cardiologist at the Charing Cross Hospital in London, invited Clare Maxwell-Hudson, a therapist who has developed her own system of massage, to offer her massage therapy to some of his patients. There were measurable falls in blood pressure and decreased anxiety levels. Since then, other health professionals, including nurses and doctors, have begun to incorporate massage into their practice.

Further reading

– Jackson, A. 1993. *Massage Therapy*. London: Macdonald Optima.

What is massage?

Massage is a manual technique which uses a variety of strokes to move the muscles and soft tissue of the body. The movements break up the fibrous tissue, loosen stiff joints, and clear the joints and tissue of acids and deposits. The massage strokes can also affect the circulatory, lymphatic and nervous systems.

By rubbing, stroking, tapping and kneading, a therapist aims to relieve the tensions held in the body of her or his client. Massage first alleviates pain, then works on rebalancing the affected area and strengthening it. Massage is more than physical manipulation, however: like any form of touch, massage also brings with it warmth and comfort through the physical contact with another.

Massage techniques

Various massage techniques have been developed, but all include certain common rhythmic movements (Box 3.1).

BOX 3.1
BASIC MASSAGE STROKES

Effleurage (Figure 3.1)
Types and methods

- *General effleurage* Both hands are placed flat on the area to be massaged, and are moved slowly over it in a gliding motion using gentle pressure.
- *Circling* The flats of both hands are moved in broad overlapping circles over the area to be massaged.
- *Feathering* The fingertips brush lightly over the area to be massaged.

When to use effleurage

In making contact with the person being massaged and in breaking contact after a massage; to spread the oil or talc at the start of a massage; to find out where the tension is; to relax, reassure and sedate the client; to make the whole body feel part of the massage experience.

Deeper-pressure strokes
Types and methods

- *Petrissage* The thumbs, fingers or heels of the hand can be used to make deeper strokes (Figure 3.2).
- *Friction* The tops of fingers or thumbs can be used to move tissue under the skin by using small circular movements and gradually increasing the pressure.
- *Kneading* Both hands together, or alternately, squeeze and release the area being massaged.
- *Pulling up* Both hands, used alternately, firmly lift the area being massaged.
- *Wringing* Like a gentle 'Chinese burn', using both hands.

When to use deeper-pressure strokes

To relax muscles deeply, to improve blood and lymphatic circulation, to help break up and dispose of waste products; to work on bony parts and joints. Kneading and stretching are particularly good for relaxing the soft fleshy parts of the body such as the buttocks.

Tapotement (Figure 3.3)
Types and methods

- *Hacking* Rhythmic chopping movements with the side of the hand. The wrist should be relaxed.

- *Cupping* Hands are cupped to form a hollow and then brought down alternately on the area to be massaged. This traps air against the skin and should sound like horses' hooves.
- *Tapping* Tapping is done with the pads of the fingers.

When to use tapotement

These percussive strokes stimulate circulation and the nervous system. They also stimulate soft tissue and tone the skin.

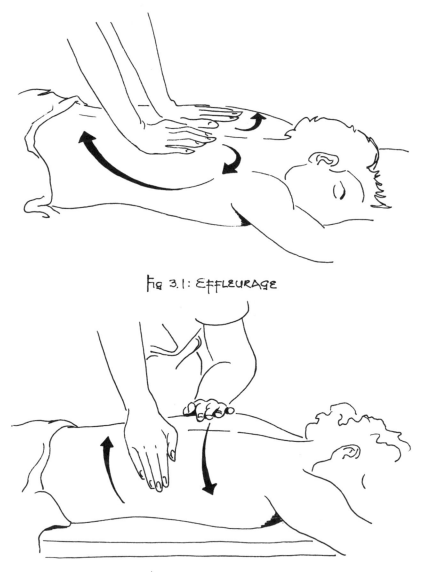

Fig 3.1: EFFLEURAGE

Fig 3.2: PETRISSAGE

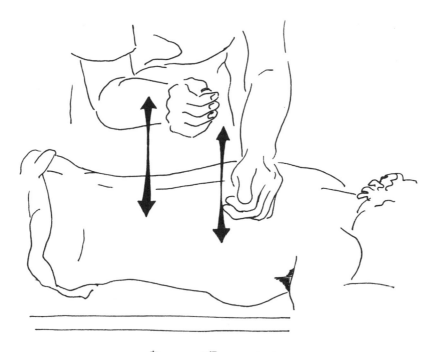

Fig 3.3 : Tapotement

Each movement is said to have a different effect, and a massage therapist will select the most appropriate for his or her client. What part of the body is massaged depends on the client's needs. In some cases a whole body massage may be offered (which will take about an hour), in others simply the neck and shoulders (perhaps ten minutes). Someone who is very ill may have only their hands or feet massaged.

Some therapists will give a massage on a **treatment couch**, while others prefer to work on the floor. All will ensure that the treatment room and their hands are warm, as clients will usually undress to some degree. It is important to help the client to relax and therapists will ensure that the client's body is not unnecessarily exposed.

Most therapists will use a **pure oil** when massaging, and if they have had appropriate additional training, will add **essential oils** to this (see Chapter 6).

A massage should be a pleasant experience, but some practitioners believe that a certain amount of pain may be necessary in order to release tensions in the body. Clients should always feel able to discuss how much pain they are able to take, and to express their own preferences about how vigorous a massage they prefer.

Types of massage

Therapeutic massage forms the basis of many other therapies, including acupressure, aromatherapy, the metamorphic technique, reflexology, and shiatsu.

There are also different types of therapeutic massage, each of which places a different emphasis on different elements of the therapy. **Intuitive massage**, for example, emphasises the importance of 'getting in touch' with the client's tensions and emotional state. **Holistic massage** places the treatment within a holistic framework; the therapist will emphasise the importance of looking at her or his client's lifestyle, as well as offering a massage for a particular problem.

Gerda Boyesen, a Norwegian psychologist, physiotherapist and Reichian analyst, has developed another type of therapeutic massage – **biodynamic massage** – which is based on Reichian principles. The body, she argues, can resolve emotional traumas and shocks if it is helped, through massage, to relieve itself of its patterns of chronic tension and blocks. Each organ, according to Boyesen, has two functions, one physical and one esoteric; the esoteric function of the intestine, for example, is to digest stress. Using a stethoscope to listen to the noises inside the abdomen, Boyesen argues that it is possible to distinguish the noises which denote that emotional energy has be set free.

Swedish massage is not, as some would have us believe, the stuff of massage parlours. It is a scientific system of therapeutic massage developed by Per Hendrik Ling, based on sound anatomical and physiological principles. Most forms of massage use some of the techniques from Swedish massage.

Further reading

- Downing, G. 1989. *The Massage Book*. London: Arkana.
- Jackson, A. 1993. *Massage Therapy*. London: Macdonald Optima.
- Maxwell-Hudson, C. 1988. *The Complete Massage Book*. London: Dorling Kindersley.

Indications

Massage is associated primarily with relieving stress by relaxing the muscles and hence the body. In this context it is therefore thought to be helpful for many stress-related conditions, including insomnia; headaches caused by the constriction of a blood vessel due to muscle spasm; and backache, if due to muscle spasm (if the pain is due to spinal problems, massage is contra-indicated).

As massage has demonstrable physiological effects on the systems of the body, there is a wide range of conditions that therapists claim they can treat successfully. These include high blood pressure; arthritic and rheumatic pain; symptoms of asthma; back pain; symptoms of colds; constipation; depression; muscular strain; sciatic pain; and pain from varicose veins.

The technique of manual lymph drainage is thought to help the body get rid of waste substances faster and is therefore useful in various disorders, especially those involving swelling or injury, fluid retention, and acne or eczema.

Massage is regularly used within the field of sports to help prevent and to treat injuries.

Massage is a useful preventive therapy and a health-promoting therapy. It is thought, for example, to be able to improve muscle tone and to reduce muscular atrophy due to forced in inactivity. Some therapists claim that regular massage will improve eyesight and hearing, halt and reverse the balding process, and lessen wrinkles (by improving the circulation).

Claims have also been made that massage helps reduce cellulite. The London College of Massage (see 'Resources'), for example, has set up a cellulite clinic which treats the problem from a holistic perspective.

Babies also are thought to benefit from massage. There have been suggestions that baby massage aids respiration, digestion, circulation, and the nervous system; and that it may be a key to reducing infant mortality rates. Many common childhood ailments, it is claimed, can be successfully treated with massage, including colic, diarrhoea, coughs, colds, and constipation.

Baby massage, if performed by the mother, also reinforces the relationship between the child and the mother, and should contribute to the baby's sense of well-being.

BOX 3.2
USING MASSAGE

Simple neck and shoulder massage

This massage sequence can be done through clothes. The person receiving the massage should sit in a chair which leaves the upper back and neck free.

Stand behind the chair and gently make contact with the receiver's shoulders using the heel of your hand. Gently push your hand into the shoulder and squeeze the muscles. Using your own body weight, lean your thumbs into the shoulder muscles between the spine and the shoulder blade and rotate your thumbs.

Then, holding the receiver's forehead in one hand, lean into and squeeze the neck muscles, including the base of the skull, with your other hand. Next move your arm so that it is across the receiver's chest to provide support, and use the heel of your other hand to massage the upper back and shoulders. To increase the pressure you exert, lean into the shoulders as you do this. Then gently rotate each of the receiver's arms. To finish the massage, stroke the receiver's forehead, head, and down the back; and squeeze the arms gently. Finish by resting your hands on the shoulders.

You can then stroke down the receiver's legs and hold his or her feet for a few seconds as a way of incorporating the rest of the body into the massage you have just completed.

Simple hand massage

First make sure the receiver is sitting comfortably and that you can work on his or her hands easily. This sequence can be performed with or without oil. If oil is used, take care with the receiver's clothes: roll up his or her sleeves and place a towel under the hands.

Gently take one hand and massage around the wrist with your thumbs. Then hold the receiver's hand palm up and stroke the palm with the heel of your hands. Lean your thumbs into the area and circle over it.

Then turn the hand over and support it with the fingers of both your hands while you stroke the back of the receiver's hand with your thumbs. Squeeze between the bones on the back of the hand, and, gently but firmly, squeeze, wring and stretch each finger in turn. Complete the massage by gently stroking the receiver's shoulders, arms and hands.

Self-massage

For backache

Lie on your back on the floor or a firm surface and bring your knees up to your chest. Then gently rock backwards and forwards for one minute. Sit up, and press your fingers firmly into the top of your buttocks and push them in four times. Repeat this all round the top of your buttocks and on either side of your lower spine.

For headaches

First press your index and middle finger of each hand into the bottom of the occipital bone at the base of your head. You should hold this position for seven seconds, and repeat three times. Then, using the same fingers, press them on your temples and make circular movements in both directions.

Contra-indications

Massage is generally a very safe, relaxing and rejuvenating therapy. There are, however, some guidelines which should be followed to avoid endangering patients.

The following contra-indications (valid for shiatsu as well as massage) are not intended to be comprehensive and advice should always be taken from a more experienced colleague or a professional massage therapist if there is any doubt about whether massage is an appropriate treatment for a particular patient.

Massage should not be undertaken in the following situations:

- If the client has eaten within two hours, has an infectious disease (including infectious skin diseases), high fever, or acute inflammation.
- If the client has a serious health problem such as heart disease or cancer, or has recently undergone surgery (unless consent from the appropriate consultant has been given).
- If the client is in the first three months of pregnancy. Massage should be given with great care during the rest of the pregnancy, avoiding the ankles, the lower back and the pelvic areas. This is because the internal organs may be tender and very active, and vigorous massage may cause disruption or injury. It is also advisable to avoid abdominal massage if a woman is menstruating, for the same reasons.

The following should also be taken into consideration:

- Scar tissue, varicose veins, bruising, tender or inflamed areas, and sites of recent fractures should not be massaged directly.
- Clients should not drink alcohol or take non-prescription drugs before or straight after a massage.
- Do not massage for too long – a whole body massage rarely takes more than one hour. It is important to avoid massaging one area for too long, to prevent tissue damage.

Further reading

- Dawes, N. & F. Harrold, 1990. *Massage Cures*. London: Thorsons.
- Jackson, A. 1993. *Massage Therapy*. London: Macdonald Optima.
- Tlinen, J. & M. Cash 1988. *Sports Massage*. London: Stanley Paul.

Research

That touch is beneficial has been shown in a variety of studies (Montague 1971). The value of massage has also been investigated. Here are some examples.

In cancer care

In a study of 513 cancer patients, 243 relatives and 143 bereaved relatives who were referred to four cancer support nurses in North Lancashire and South Lakeland between January 1990 and January 1991. Some 32 per cent of the patients, 12 per cent of the relatives, and 49 per cent of the bereaved relatives used relaxation therapy, of which massage was the main preference. Between 68 and 74 per cent of patients (depending on which type of relaxation therapy was chosen) said they had benefited from the therapy.

– McIllmurray, M. B. & P. E. Holdcroft 1993. Supportive care and the use of relaxation therapy in a district cancer service. *British Journal of Cancer* 67: 861–4.

With premature babies

Premature babies given three 15-minute massages during three consecutive hours per day for ten days averaged a 21 per cent weight gain per day (35 g cf. 28 g), and were discharged five days earlier. Forty babies had been assigned to either the treatment or the control groups for this study.

– Scafidi, F. S., T. M. Field, S. M. Schanberg, *et al*. 1990. Massage stimulates growth in preterm infants: a replication. *Infant Behaviour and Development* 13: 167–88.

With depressed children and adolescents

In a study of 52 hospitalised, depressed and adjustment-disorder children and adolescents, those who received a daily 30-minute back massage over a five-day period were less depressed and anxious and had lower saliva cortisol levels than the control group who simply viewed relaxing videotapes. Nurses also reported that night-time sleep improved among the massage groups, and the urinary cortisol and norepinephrine (noradrenaline) levels decreased among the depressed patients who received massage.

– Field, T., C. Morrow, C. Valdeon, *et al*. 1992. Massage reduces anxiety in child and adolescent psychiatric patients. *Journal of the American Academy of Childhood and Adolescent Psychiatry* 31(1): 125–31.

With the elderly

Twenty-one residents (17 women and 4 men) participated in this study. They were randomly allocated to three groups, those who received 'back massage with normal conversation', those who received 'conversation only', and the last group who received 'no intervention'. According to the researchers:

With the exception of mean diastolic blood pressure which showed no change from pre-test to post-test and heart rate which increased from post-test to delayed time interval, there was a statistically insignificant decrease in mean scores on all variables (the Spielberger Self-Evaluation Questionnaire – to test anxiety levels, electromyographic recordings, and systolic blood pressure) in the back massage group from pre-test to post-test and from post-test to delayed time interval. There was a statistically significant difference in the mean anxiety (STAI) score between the back massage group and the no intervention group. The difference between the back massage group and the conversation only group approached statistical significance.

The participants said they thought the back massage was relaxing.

- Fraser, J. & J. R. Kerr, 1993. Psychophysiological effects of back massage on elderly institutionalized patients. *Journal of Advanced Nursing* 18: 238–45.

With people receiving radiotherapy

This pilot study examined the effects of gentle back massage on the perceived well-being of six female patients receiving radiotherapy for breast cancer. Pre- and post-intervention measures of symptom distress and mood were made, using the subjects themselves as their own controls. The patients reported less symptom distress, higher degrees of tranquillity and vitality, and less tension and tiredness following the back massage, when compared with the control intervention (10-minute rest period instead of a 10-minute massage).

- Sims, S. 1986. Slow stroke back massage for cancer patients. *Nursing Times* 82(13): 47–50.

Other research

A review of other research into massage can be found in the following article by Mario-Paul Cassar:

- Cassar, M.-P. 1993. Massage is the medium. *The Therapist* (Spring 1993), 1(1): 30–1.

Other studies which have investigated the therapeutic effects of massage include:

- Avakyan, G. N. 1990. Pressure and massage therapy to relieve fatigue. *Advanced Clinical Care* (September–October), 5(5): 10–11.
- Kampschroeder, F. 1990. Trigger point and transfrictional massage: a case report. *Chiropractic* (July), 6(2): 40–2.
- Li, Y. 1990. Facial cosmetic massage. *Journal of Traditional Chinese Medicine* (September), 10(3): 219–21.

- Puustjarvi, K. 1990. The effects of massage in patients with chronic tension headache. *Acupuncture and Electrotherapy Research* **15**(2): 159–62.
- Shao, X. 1990. Effect of massage and temperature on the permeability of initial lymphatics. *Lymphology* **23**(1): 48–50.

Implications for nursing

'Touching and soothing is integral to nursing' says massage therapist Clare Maxwell-Hudson, who designed the massage module taught at the Royal College of Nursing's Institute of Advanced Nursing Education (see 'Resources'). She argues that 'a nurse with massage skills will have a better quality of communication in his or her touch; will soothe and relax the patient and transmit a sense of care in a matter of minutes; you don't always have to find time for a more formal massage' (Anon 1993).

Massage is potentially of value to a wide range of patients and is already being used in many units, wards, and clinics in the UK, as more and more nurses, midwives and health visitors add this skill to their list of qualifications.

Massage therapists are also happy to offer their services to the NHS. However, such offers are not always welcomed, as the following account from one massage therapist – who had contacted many different hospitals – reveals (Crawley 1992):

> I did have one apparent breakthrough. The director sounded very keen, and put me in touch with the manager of services and the senior sister. After an exchange of letters I had two interviews which ended with a virtual offer of a part-time position with the transplant unit.
>
> I was shown around the unit and introduced to the staff, even shown the place from which I would work. The agreement implied my starting with six hours a week paid (at a rate of about £6 an hour) and putting in an additional 10 hours of voluntary work (my offer). I was given personal application forms to fill in, as well as a health screening.
>
> Because of the paperwork involved, and the need to inform the nurses at their regular meeting, we agreed that I would start four weeks later. As the time approached and no written confirmation details came, I contacted the senior sister – and discovered that the whole thing had been reversed.
>
> I was given the impression that the nurses were not keen to have me there as a paid practitioner, rather that they should be trained to provide such services as massage. The only option I was left with was that of being 'on call' with my services offered in the same way as those of the hairdresser or aromatherapist (and as the latter offered her services voluntarily I was told there was little chance of my getting paid for mine).

It is a pity that such situations occur, as patients are potentially being denied access to the services of a professionally trained practitioner as a result of territorial disputes by nurses. While it is laudable that nurses wish to receive training themselves, is it right to deny patients the service until such time as the nurses complete their training, if indeed their hospital gives them the go-ahead to undertake it?

In 1993 the National Association of Health Authorities and Trusts published the results of a national survey (NAHAT 1993) of purchasers which examined their attitudes towards the availability of complementary therapies within the NHS. More than 70 per cent of family health services authorities (FHSAs) and GP fund-holders (GPFHs), and 65 per cent of district health authorities (DHAs), were in favour of some or all complementary therapies being available on the NHS – that is, free at the point of contact. Nine health-promotion clinics which offered massage had been given approval by FHSAs.

Massage is also a relaxation technique that nurses can offer to each other. For example, a 5-minute neck and shoulder massage may release tensions and pains which were making a shift seem twice as long, or a gentle face massage may avert a headache at the end of a shift. A weekend course may be all that is necessary to offer this sort of help to colleagues.

Alternatively, massage therapists are often prepared to visit units to offer massage to staff. For example, massage therapist Marcia Kenny offers massage to people working with cancer patients at the Royal Marsden Hospital in London. She says, 'Of the staff I see some come for massage because it makes them feel good . . . Others come with physical symptoms, back pain, stiff necks, headaches and tight shoulders, and generally feel low. As they begin to relax and offload it soon becomes clear that many are suffering from all the normal anxieties of life' (Kenny 1992).

However, nurses wanting to start incorporating massage into the care given to patients should undertake a thorough training as there are many circumstances under which massage is contra-indicated and is therefore potentially dangerous to patients. As health professionals, nurses are accountable for their actions and should be able to demonstrate that they are competent practitioners. The *Code of Professional Conduct* also demands such competence of nurses.

Examples of the use of massage in nursing and health care

In intensive care

Caroline Stevensen, an intensive-care sister at the Middlesex Hospital in London, trained as a massage therapist. She has introduced massage on her unit with good results, and helps train nurses from the health authority in massage.

– Stevensen, C. 1992. Holistic Power. *Nursing Times* **88**(38): 68–70.

In the care of the dying

Rosemary Byass, staff nurse at Mount Edgcumbe Hospice in St Austell, offered massage to patients at the hospice. In her *Nursing Times* article she says, 'Anyone concerned with the care of the dying, whether within or outside the medical team, should learn the techniques of massage. It is a beneficial, holistic and harmless means of helping patients "live until they die", and it only requires empathy and a pair of hands.

– Byass, R. 1988. Soothing body and soul. *Nursing Times* **84**(24): 39–41.

At Milestone House, a purpose-built AIDS hospice in Edinburgh, complementary therapies are offered to residents. According to the hospice's manager, Ruth Murie, 'the nature of the disease means people often choose therapies such as massage for relaxation rather than take a tablet, as they are often already taking a large amount of medication'.

– Murie, R. A milestone in care. *Nursing Times* **88**(42): 24–7.

In bowel management

Physiotherapist Marian Emly has successfully used abdominal massage with clients who have cerebral palsy, as an effective treatment for constipation. Other health professionals, including nurses, have used abdominal massage to help with such problems as faecal incontinence and constipation in elderly patients.

– Emly, M. 1993. Abdominal massage. *Nursing Times* **89**(3): 34–6.

In health visiting

Gill Thornton is a health visitor working in Wickham. She trained at the London College of Massage and offers massage treatments privately, and occasionally as a health visitor. Patients are referred to her by a GP. She has taught baby massage at antenatal classes and as a relaxation technique. She has also treated two women for postnatal depression.

In general practice

Jackie Pietroni is a nurse tutor, but also trained in massage at the Clare Maxwell-Hudson School of Massage. She has a massage clinic at her husband's GP surgery in Ealing, as part of the surgery's health-promotion initiatives. Patients are offered four consecutive weekly sessions, each of half an hour – a stipulation of the FHSA. Her patients include a man who had had a coronary artery bypass graft; stressed executives; patients with aching legs, stiff necks and shoulders; and pregnant women, new mothers, and a woman embarking on an IVF programme.

– Pietroni, J. 1991. NHS funds GP massage clinic. *Massage* (Autumn 1991): 1.

With people with anorexia

Superintendent physiotherapist Kirstie Davison has used massage with patients with anorexia at the Mental Health Unit in Coney Hill Hospital, Gloucester. She says massage can be used to 'encourage the patient with a distorted body image to feel "in touch" with herself.'

– Davison, K. 1990. Reaching out to anorexic patients. *Therapy Weekly* 17(18): 4.

Resources

Equipment

A treatment couch or a single futon will be needed in order to treat patients outside of a ward setting, plus several large soft towels to cover the patient and the surface she or he is lying on, and plenty of cushions which the patient can then use to make herself or himself comfortable.

Training and regulation

Massage can be offered at different levels, from that of the beauty therapist at a salon or health club to that of the massage therapist who works with people who are ill.

It is possible for anyone to learn the basic massage strokes, and there are many weekend courses for beginners. After completing such a course you can certainly practise on family and friends, but it is unwise to start using your newly-acquired skills on sick patients. To train properly can take a year or more. The best-known training qualification is ITEC (International Therapy Examination Council). Many schools and therapists feel that the ITEC standard is too low, however, and courses offering the ITEC qualification can vary enormously in length and quality.

There is no formal regulation of massage therapists in the UK. However, in September 1992 the British Massage Therapy Council was formed. It is, says a spokesman, likely to affiliate formally with the umbrella organisation, the British Complementary Medicine Association (see Chapter 1). If and when this occurs, members will be subject to the BCMA's codes of conduct and ethics, and will be able to enjoy the benefits of its insurance scheme.

Massage associations and colleges have been able to join the Council since January 1993. It is the intention of the Council to improve training standards and it is keen to investigate National Vocational Qualifications as an alternative to ITEC.

For more information on the Council, write to:

British Massage Therapy Council (BMTC)
c/o 9 Elm Road, Worthing, West Sussex BN11 1PG.

As far as nurses are concerned, massage is one of the therapies that has been included in the first course jointly accredited by the Royal College of Nursing's Institute of Advanced Nursing Education and the Institute for Complementary Medicine (see Chapter 1). This course is part of a module for a degree from the University of Manchester. It takes a year and is a 50-hour module. It is not a professional massage course, but is designed specifically for the nursing profession.

Some Project 2000 courses and some nursing degree and diploma courses are also introducing massage as part of their curricula. For example, at the Oxford Brookes University's School of Health Care Studies, one of the nurse teacher-counsellors, Theresa Bentley, has introduced a series of workshops in massage for nurses as part of a module on aspects of therapeutic caring, after training at the Clare Maxwell-Hudson School of Massage. Some of the student nurses have gone on to do a three-month ITEC training course in massage in their own time. The hope is to make the study of massage part of formal nurse training on the modular course at Oxford.

The Institute for Complementary Medicine's British Register of Complementary Practitioners has a massage division, and a list of these practitioners is available from the ICM.

Useful addresses

The following list is not comprehensive, but may be helpful in finding out about available courses.

Allied School of Remedial Massage (ASRM)
37 Barnfield Close, Galmpton, Brixham, Devon TQ5 OLY.

Centre for Massage and Movement Studies (CMMS)
17 Beechdale Road, London SW2 2BN.

Clare Maxwell-Hudson School of Massage (CMHSM)
PO Box 457, London NW2 4BR.

The school also has an association for graduates of the school: The Massage Therapy Institute of Great Britain. This has a register of practitioners (currently about 600), and an insurance scheme for practitioners. The Institute is affiliated with other massage organisations. For more information, write to: PO Box 2726, London NW2 3NR.

College of Holistic Medicine (CHM)
4 Craigpark, Glasgow G31 2NA.

Fellowship of Sports Masseurs and Therapists School of Sports Massage (FSMTSSM)
66 Hillfield Park, Winchmore Hill, London N21 3QL.

Gerda Boyesen Centre for Biodynamic Psychology and Psychotherapy (GBCBPP)
Acacia House, Centre Avenue, Acton Park, London W3 7JX.

London College of Massage (LCM)
5–6 Newman Passage, London W1P 3PF.

Practitioners qualifying from the College can go onto the British Register of Complementary Practitioners, which is managed by the ICM. The college is also a member of the Association of Physical and Natural Therapists, which has a register and a code of conduct, and which offers insurance.

Northern Institute of Massage (NIM)
100 Waterloo Road, Blackpool, Lancashire FY4 1AW.

This is the oldest school of massage in the UK. A register of practitioners trained by the Institute is available. Graduates of the Institute became members of the London and Counties Society of Physiologists and must therefore abide by the Society's code of conduct.

Sussex School of Massage (SSM)
26 Victoria Street, Brighton BN1 3FQ.

West London School of Therapeutic Massage (WLSTM)
41a St Luke's Road, London W11 1DD.

Which training course?

It is worth contacting the BMTC, the RCN and the ICM to find out what courses they recommend, particularly as this complementary therapy is largely unregulated and there is no one organisation that has a comprehensive list of accredited schools.

Recommended reading

- Dawes, N. & F. Harrold, 1990. *Massage Cures*. London: Thorsons.
- Downing, G. 1989. *The Massage Book*. London: Arkana.
- Lidell, L. 1992. *The Book of Massage*. London: Ebury Press.
- Maxwell-Hudson, C. 1988. *The Complete Massage Book*. London: Dorling Kindersley.
- Tlinen, J. & M. Cash 1988. *Sports Massage*. London: Stanley Paul.

References

- Anon 1993. Royal College of Nursing now has massage therapy in its curriculum. *The Therapist* (Spring 1993), 1(1): 6–7.
- Crawley, E. 1992. Finding hospital placements has so far not been easy. *Massage* (Winter 1992/3), 7(3): 8.
- Kenny, M. 1992. Taking care of the carers. *Massage* (Winter 1992/3), 7(3):9.
- Montague, A. 1971. *Touching – the human significance of the skin*. New York: Columbia University Press.
- NAHAT 1993. *Complementary Therapies in the NHS* (Research Paper No. 10). London: National Association of Health Authorities and Trusts.

4 SHIATSU

Historical background

Tao-Yinn is a system of exercises which developed in China around the 6th century BC, including massage and pressure-point manipulation, which aimed to promote the well-being of the people who practised it upon themselves. By the 6th century AD, as China and Japan came into increasingly greater contact through trade, Tao-Yinn had become integrated into Chinese medical practice, and as such, was introduced to Japanese students of healing.

Over time, a form of massage called Anma developed in Japan, incorporating many elements of Tao-Yinn; by the 16th century, Anma was an integral part of Japanese medical training. It slowly decreased in importance, however, as practitioners developed other forms of treatment; by the start of the present century, it was seen as little more than a relaxing massage technique, whose practitioners were not allowed to use it as a medical treatment.

Some of those practitioners sought to promote Anma's therapeutic value, and coined the word 'shiatsu' to get around the restrictions surrounding Anma. In 1919, a therapist called Tamai Tempaku published a book, *Shiatsu Ho*, which stimulated interest and research in the subject; growing numbers of people claimed that the treatment had many benefits, and in the mid-1950s the Japanese government accorded shiatsu recognition as a legitimate therapy, and the wheel had come full circle.

Shiatsu was not very well known in the West until the early 1960s, when practitioners started appearing in the United States, and then Europe; the therapy grew in popularity throughout the following years, and is now becoming more widely known in Britain, with the spread of classes teaching the technique, and the publication of a number of books and videos.

Further reading

- Jarmey, C. 1992. *Thorsons Introductory Guide to Shiatsu*. London: Thorsons.
- Liechti, E. 1992. *Shiatsu: Japanese massage for health and fitness*. Shaftesbury: Element.

What is shiatsu?

Shiatsu is a Japanese word, which translates as 'finger pressure'. The Japanese Ministry of Health and Welfare defines shiatsu therapy as: 'a form of manipulation administered by the thumbs, fingers and palms, without the use of any instrument, mechanical or otherwise, to apply pressure to the human skin, to correct internal malfunctioning, promote and maintain health, and treat specific diseases' (cited in Jarmey 1992).

In Japan, many households have at least one person who is proficient in shiatsu, where it is almost like a Western first-aid box. It is not just for when health fails, though: as the definition above makes plain, it is also used in health maintenance and promotion.

The therapy has a lot of appeal for health-care workers: it is apparently simple, it is non-invasive, and it shares a theoretical framework with acupuncture (see Chapter 13), which has the dual virtues of being holistic and long-established.

How it works

To understand the theory behind shiatsu, it is first necessary to examine some concepts fundamental to Oriental medicine and philosophy; a fuller discussion can be found in Chapter 13.

Ki

Ki (the Japanese word for **Qi**, a fundamental concept in traditional Chinese medicine) is energy, in the widest sense. Everything is a manifestation of Ki, from rocks to thought processes. Everything in the universe is made up of Ki, and everything is in a constant state of change, because Ki is a motive force.

Ki has two qualities, **Yin** and **Yang**; these are opposites, but neither can exist without the other. The symbol for **Yin/Yang** is a circle, signifying wholeness and infinity, divided by a curved line, which represents movement and the constant flow of Yin and Yang into each other. Within each coloured area is a dot of the opposite colour, which symbolises the coexistence of opposites within everything.

Yin is associated with darkness, coldness, immobility and calm, while Yang has the opposite associations: light, heat, movement and activity. Yin is female, and Yang is male.

Each person has a tendency to be either more Yin or more Yang in her or his nature, but a balance is usually maintained. If either Yin or Yang becomes too predominant, though, the imbalance may be manifested as signs and symptoms: too much Yin is associated with bodily coolness and lethargy, while excessive Yang causes restlessness and fevers.

Meridians

Ki is believed to circulated throughout the body, but there are several **Meridians**, or channels, where its flow is most concentrated. Meridians connect organs in the body, but, as is explained in a later section, there is a great deal of room for confusion when discussing anatomy and physiology in the terms used by practitioners of some therapies.

Where the Meridians pass near the surface, acupressure can be applied; these areas are called **acupoints**, or **tsubo**. When a channel or tsubo is judged to be 'full', the term used is **jitsu**; if it is 'empty', the term is **kyo**. Jitsu and kyo correspond to Yin and Yang; as might be expected from what has been said already about this concept, 'fullness' and 'emptiness' are relative, not absolute terms. Ki moves in a way that is best likened to fluidity, and its concentration in areas will vary, with a general harmony over the whole body; problems arise when there is an acute or chronic interruption to the flow.

Organs

It is difficult for the trained health-care worker to avoid confusion on first reading a text which refers to structures in the body in terms that do not seem to fit with what one already knows about organ function. For example, a problem with the Heart Meridian may be associated with emotional disturbances, an association which is hard to explain in physiological terms. The reason for this is apparently straightforward: in Oriental medicine, the **Organ** referred to does not just mean the physical structure, but also relates to a whole series of functions perceived to be related to it. Thus, when the 'heart' is referred to, the practitioner is talking not just about cardiac function, as a Western medical practitioner would understand it, but also about a whole range of emotional activity (which, interestingly, corresponds almost exactly to the lay understanding of 'matters of the heart'). To avoid confusion, many texts have adopted the convention of capitalising the first letter of an Organ's name – for example, Heart – when referring to it in this extended, almost metaphorical, sense.

There are two additional 'Organs': the **Heart Governor**, and the **Triple Heater**. The first of these is also referred to, using the capital-letter convention, as the **Pericardium**, or **Heart Protector**, and is considered to be concerned with the physical actions of the heart as a pump. The Triple Heater refers to three central energy centres or **chakras**, found at the levels of the heart, the solar plexus, and the **tanden** (an area three fingers' width below the umbilicus). Each Heater is connected with the Organs in its vicinity; the Triple Heater as a whole acts as the body's temperature regulator. Some modern writers now say that the Triple Heater is also associated with the lymphatic and immune systems.

The Five Elements

Another concept which must be understood is that of the **Five Elements** (sometimes called **Phases** or **Transformations**). This ascribes the qualities of **Metal, Water, Wood, Fire** and **Earth** to Ki in different processes of change. There are correspondences between one Element and another, and energy flows between them in cycles. Different Organs are associated with specific Elements, as are senses and emotions. (This is discussed in more detail in Chapter 13.)

Disturbances in the flow of Ki

Practitioners of shiatsu are keen to stress the preventive, or health-promoting, aspects of the treatment: an experienced practitioner can spot imbalances before they cause physical symptoms, and correct them. This does not rule out shiatsu for the treatment of an existing physical disorder, however, although there are a number of conditions for which it is not indicated, as will be discussed later.

Each Meridian is associated with an Organ, but this is not to be thought of solely as the physical structure. If there is an imbalance of Ki in any meridian, physical symptoms will result.

Disturbances in the flow of Ki come from a disturbance in the balance of Yin and Yang, and the result is a disease. In shiatsu, the presumed causes of imbalance are the same as in other branches of Oriental medicine: internal, external, or 'other'.

Internal causes

These are inseparably linked with emotions, which are, as we have seen, associated with specific Meridians. There are seven fundamental emotions: sadness; fear; worry; pensiveness; anger; overexcitement; shock or fright (note that 'shock' here is used in its lay sense). All of these emotions are normal, of course; it is only when they exceed a certain degree of intensity that they cause problems.

Sadness is thought to affect the Lungs; fear, the Kidneys; worry and pensiveness, the Spleen and Pancreas; anger, the Liver; overexcitement, the Heart; and shock or fright have a widespread effect, but chiefly on the Kidneys, the Heart, and the Small Intestine.

External causes

Climate is thought to have an effect upon the body's health, relating to the Five Elements: heat, for example, adversely affects the

Fire Element, while cold weather acts on the Water Element; dampness affects Earth; dryness affects Metal; and wind acts on Wood. Each produces symptoms affecting the related Organs.

Other causes

This category includes just about every other possible reason for the appearance of symptoms, including stress, the level of physical activity, trauma, toxic substances (both natural, such as bee stings, and synthetic, such as some drugs), and 'constitution', which may be used as shorthand for an expression of how much Ki an individual has 'in reserve'.

Visiting a shiatsu practitioner

Each session lasts for up to an hour. The first session is taken up with a health assessment; the practitioner uses visual and verbal clues and information gained from the client about past and present health, lifestyle, family history, and so on, to build up an overall picture of the person he or she will be treating.

A physical assessment is then carried out, in which the shiatsu practitioner 'feels' the quality of Ki within the person, by touching areas of the torso. By its very nature, it is quite subjective; this is how one practitioner explains it:

Experienced practitioners can feel blocked, overactive or insufficient Ki within any area of the body, because it reflects in a certain 'quality' or 'response' to touch. This is particularly clear when working directly on any of the fourteen channels through which Ki circulates. Where too much Ki causes a blockage along a Channel, the blocked Ki feels like a swelling from which Ki is trying to break out. It feels 'active' and 'hard' in the same way as an over-inflated balloon feels hard; the more you press it, the more it resists. It may not present as an actual swelling, but will definitely feel energetically confined and under pressure. As with a balloon, you would not want to press it too hard for fear of an explosion. An explosion of pain accompanies pressure which is too direct and heavy upon the blocked area ... Insufficient Ki in an area makes that area feel empty, lifeless and devoid of zest. It ... may well feel soft, lacking resilience. It may also feel hard, but not the hardness of an inflated balloon or car tyre – this is the hardness of inert matter such as the dried-out crust on top of a stale loaf of bread. Contrast this with a loaf of bread just out of the oven, which has the Ki of freshness and warmth to give it some bounce.

(Jarmey 1992.)

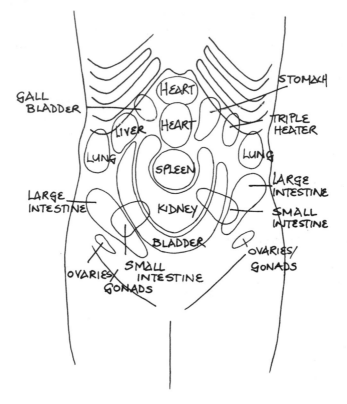

Fig 4.1 : The Hara and its Diagnostic Areas

There are two areas on the torso which the shiatsu practitioner can use to aid in formulating a diagnosis. One is the **hara**, on the abdomen (Figure 4.1); the second area covers most of the back. Information can also be gathered by feeling pulses at six positions on each wrist, while the tongue and face also have diagnostic potential (Figure 4.2).

Diagnostic touch is always carried out through a layer of clothing, preferably a single one of natural fibre. Practitioners find that they can 'feel' below the skin surface better in this way, and there are other advantages: treatment can be given anywhere, and the potential problems associated with a professional relationship where the client is partially unclothed are less likely to arise.

The assessment can be carried out in a sitting position, but treatment is likely to be carried out with the client lying down. There are three techniques: tonification, dispersal, and calming.

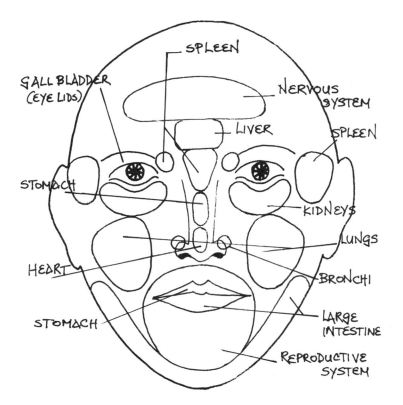

Fig 4.2: DIAGNOSTIC AREAS OF THE FACE

Tonification

This is sustained pressure, delivered at right angles to the body, which is intended to increase the circulation of both blood and energy in an area.

Dispersal

There are several techniques included under 'dispersal', all of which involve active movement such as stretching and squeezing. As the name suggests, the aim is to break up a blockage of blood or energy.

Calming

There is little or no pressure in 'calming', which can consist of a simple holding or gentle rocking movement. This is intended to counteract agitated energy.

The key to successful treatment is efficient use of the therapist's body weight and position, which should be almost effortless.

Indications

As shiatsu is such a potent reliever of stress, it is of value to any person at any time, but when a health problem may be stress-related – as so many are – the therapy is particularly useful. Insomnia and headaches are often responsive to shiatsu.

Disorders of the gastro-intestinal tract, including diarrhoea, constipation, indigestion, and stomach cramp, are all conditions which practitioners feel they can alleviate, while a whole range of muscular problems may benefit from the therapy.

One well-documented area is treatment of nausea, whether caused by motion, pregnancy, or drugs; this is discussed below, under 'Research'.

There are very few health problems with which shiatsu can offer no help; more detailed information can be found in the books listed under 'Recommended reading'.

Contra-indications

Shiatsu practitioners have lists of conditions which their treatment would not help, ones where treatment is impractical, and others where matters could possibly be worsened. In the first group, acute fevers and burns are listed; in the second, contagious diseases are an obvious category.

A primary aim of the therapy is increasing the blood flow within the body, so where there is a risk of haemorrhage, or where thrombosis is suspected, shiatsu should probably be avoided. For the same reason, some practitioners recommend extreme caution when there may be a tumour in the area to be treated.

Because a degree of pressure is used, the same cautions noted in the previous chapter on massage should be observed: when the person has osteoporosis, or if there has been any recent tissue damage, inflammation, or fractures, particular care must be taken before applying pressure to any part of the body that has been affected.

If a person has high blood pressure or epilepsy, some points on the skull should be avoided.

Pregnancy is another difficult case, for although mothers-to-be may enjoy the relaxation engendered by shiatsu, there are some pressure points on the leg which practitioners say can, if manipulated, increases the chance of miscarriage.

There are many conditions which shiatsu has no direct part in treating, but when the experience of touch alone might be beneficial for the patient – for example, neoplasm and AIDS.

Research

There is very little published research on shiatsu, but because of the many similarities in their underlying theory between this therapy and acupuncture, much of the research into traditional Chinese medicine (particularly acupressure) can be used to examine the claims.

One area that has received a lot of attention is the use of 'acupressure bands' in the treatment of nausea. The theory is that there is a point on the Pericardium Meridian, found on the inside of the wrist – Pericardium 6, also referred to as P6 or *Nei Kuan* – which, if pressed, will directly suppress nausea. The acupressure bands are elasticated, and a small stud on the inner surface is thus held above the P6 point. If nausea is felt, pressure can be applied. Several studies have been carried out to see whether the effect is real or not, and the results have tended to be positive (see Box 4.1).

A leading teacher of shiatsu in this country, when looking at an early draft of this chapter, said: 'All the research relates to P6, which is a shame. It is akin to implying that all there is of interest to research in nursing is the effectiveness of applying on Elastoplast to a graze. Unfortunately, that *does* seem to be the extent of the research on shiatsu.'

With thalamic pain: a pilot study

In 1991 and 1992, a small pilot study was carried out by a shiatsu practitioner in Oxford. Thirteen people with thalamic pain were approached, and asked if they would participate in some research; seven consented, but only two went through with it. Three other people were already receiving shiatsu for thalamic pain. Of these five, three felt that shiatsu had helped, while two felt worse; as the researcher points out, thalamic pain can be worsened by touch.

Further details about this study can be obtained from the Shiatsu Society (see 'Resources').

With gynaecological surgery

From the patients admitted to a Buckinghamshire hospital for major gynaecological surgery, 40 females were paired with controls for age and surgical procedure. The members of each pair were randomised either to wear acupressure bands and to receive antiemetics as clinically indicated, or antiemetics alone.

Full data were available on 28 index patients and their controls. Those patients who wore acupressure bands needed 15.5 per cent fewer doses of antiemetics, and there was a significantly reduced level of nausea and vomiting in this group.

– Phillips, K. & L. Gill, 1993. A point of pressure. *Nursing Times* **89**(45), 44–5.

BOX 4.1
APPLYING P6 PRESSURE

Four studies in recent years have demonstrated the effectiveness of applying pressure to a point on the Pericardium Meridian.

The incidence of morning sickness was greatly reduce in 350 pregnant women in a Belfast hospital, when pressure was applied to P6.

– Dundee, J., G. Ghaley, P. F. Bell, *et al.* 1988. P6 acupressure reduces morning sickness. *Journal of the Royal Society of Medicine* **81**: 456–8.

An American trial found acupressure bands relieved morning sickness in 12 out of the 16 pregnant women studied, and improved mental well-being was reported during the periods they were worn.

– Hyde, E. 1989. Acupressure therapy for morning sickness. *Journal of Nurse-Midwifery* **34**(4): 171–7.

In a trial at Truro's Royal Cornwall Hospital, involving 18 people receiving chemotherapy for cancer (a treatment which can cause severe nausea), acupressure bands reduced the ill-effects in many of the patients, allowing them to eat and drink better.

– Stannard, D. 1989. Pressure prevents nausea. *Nursing Times* **85**(4): 33–4.

A Hampshire study of 38 patients receiving chemotherapy, where half the group wore the bands on the ankle, found a significant decrease in nausea, and improvements in mood, in those who wore the bands in the correct position.

– Price, H., G. Lewith, & C. Williams 1991. Acupressure as an antiemetic in cancer chemotherapy. *Complementary Medical Research* **5**(2): 93–4.

Implications for nursing

Training in shiatsu takes several years, part-time, but the basics are reasonably simple, and can be practised on oneself without too much trouble, providing the cautions given above are heeded.

Before embarking on administering shiatsu, nurses should have attended some form of practically-based study course, run by a member of the register of the Shiatsu Society. The risks may be small, but they are no less real for that.

Equipment: Apart from a comfortable resting place for the patient (usually a futon), the only tools used by a shiatsu practitioner are the hands and the five senses. However, because of the nature of the therapy, two things must be available: time and privacy. Any benefits of shiatsu are undermined, and possibly lost, if treatment sessions are disturbed by interruptions, or risk abrupt curtailment.

As with massage therapy, shiatsu calls for a closer degree of physical contact than many people might find comfortable, and this must always be borne in mind.

As shiatsu becomes more popular – which appears likely, because of its apparent simplicity, and the fact that a number of books and videos are available which give detailed instruction on how to administer the treatment – growing numbers of patients and clients may ask nurses, midwives and health visitors about its benefits. For this reason, it seems worth some time and effort for health-care professionals to try and familiarise themselves with the basics of the therapy, in order to be able to give informed advice, and to know where people seeking more information should be directed.

It seems that nurses who have undergone a recognised training course in this therapy might have a lot to offer patients in their care, as shiatsu is relatively safe and offers relief from many of the conditions which, if not directly responsible for the health-care problem that made nursing care necessary, can significantly affect progress.

Examples of the use of shiatsu in nursing and health care

At the time of writing, no accounts have appeared in the nursing press of nurses using shiatsu in practice. No doubt reports of nurses' practical experience with this therapy will be published in the near future.

Resources

Training and regulation

There are several different types of shiatsu, which lay emphasis on different areas. They include Namikoshi-style, which is rooted in a Western-style approach to physiology; Zen shiatsu, which proposes a more complex network of Meridians than that taught in the 'traditional' schools; and Tsubo Therapy, which is more closely related to acupuncture in its concentration on specific points on the body. There are other variants, but the aims of each are the same: to revitalise the body and mind through the use of finger pressure on the body. Unlike some therapies, though, it is not considered a disadvantage to be familiar with more than one of these variants – the Shiatsu Society, in fact, encourages it.

It is possible to attend classes which give a basic grounding in shiatsu for use on oneself, but, as might be expected, training as a practitioner is a more lengthy procedure.

The Shiatsu Society was established in 1981, and now acts as an information service for the public, and as a professional organisation for practitioners. The Society maintains a register of members who have completed a recognised course of training (minimum length: three years); having met the criteria of the school, they must then satisfy the Society's assessment panel of their abilities in theory and practice. Having done this, members may use the letters MRSS (Member of the Register of the Shiatsu Society) after their name.

A list of registered practitioners, and details of training courses, can be obtained from:

Shiatsu Society (SS)
5 Foxcote, Wokingham, Berkshire RG11 3PG.

Recommended reading

- Jarmey, C. & G. Mojay 1991. *Shiatsu – the complete guide*. London: Thorsons.
- Jarmey, C. 1992. *Thorsons' Introductory Guide to Shiatsu*. London: Thorsons.
- Liechti, E. 1992. *Shiatsu: Japanese massage for health and fitness*. Shaftesbury: Element.
- Lundberg, P. 1992. *The Book of Shiatsu*. London: Gaia.
- Moriceau, S. 1987. Shiatsu. In Stanway, A. (ed.): *The Natural Family Doctor*. London: Century.

Anyone wanting to know more about the subject can obtain a bibliography, and a list of videos, from the Shiatsu Society.

Reference

– Jarmey, C. 1992. *Thorson's Introductory Guide to Shiatsu*. London: Thorsons.

5 REFLEXOLOGY

Historical background

Although reflexology is sometimes thought of as being quite a modern therapy, most reflexology texts claim that it has a pedigree as long as that of acupuncture, making it around 5000 years old, although one text does acknowledge that 'concrete proof is evasive' (Dougans & Ellis 1992). Massage of the soles of the feet – and, more rarely, the palms of the hands – for the purposes of diagnosis and treatment of somatic disorders is claimed to have been known in China around 3000 BC, while a pictograph unearthed in Egypt, dated as originating from around 2500–2300 BC, appears to show treatment being given (Bayly 1982; Norman & Cowan 1989). Similar techniques are known to have existed in parts of India for many centuries, and there is a tradition of therapeutic foot massage among some native American tribes, although it is difficult to date the origins of the practice.

In the early 20th century, an American ear, nose and throat specialist called William H. Fitzgerald published reports of his observations that pressure on some parts of the body appeared to produce effects in other, anatomically distant areas:

> I accidentally discovered that pressure with a cotton-tipped probe on the mucocutaneous margin (where the skin joins the mucous membrane) of the nose gave an anaesthetic result as though a cocaine solution had been applied. I further found that there were many spots in the nose, mouth, throat, and on both surfaces of the tongue which, when pressed firmly, deadened definite areas of sensation. Also, that pressures exerted over any body eminence, on the hands, feet, or over the joints, produced the same characteristic results in pain relief. I found also that when pain was relieved, the condition that produced the pain was most generally relieved. This led to my 'mapping out' these various areas and their associated connections, and also noting the conditions influenced through them. This science I have named zone therapy.
>
> (Gore 1990.)

Fitzgerald's work – which was apparently first given broad publicity in a 1915 magazine article, 'To Stop That Toothache Squeeze Your Toe!' – was developed by several people, but perhaps the most influential was another American, Eunice D. Ingham. In her work throughout the 1930s, she expounded the doctrine that all parts of the body could be affected by pressure on clearly defined areas of the feet, particularly on their soles. These associated treatment techniques came to be known as the *Ingham Reflex Method of Compression Massage.*

Doreen Bayly, a student of Miss Ingham's, is widely credited as the person who did most to introduce the techniques of reflexology into Britain during the 1960s, both by opening a training school for therapists, and through her efforts to publicise the benefits of the treatment.

Reflexology has slowly and steadily increased in popularity since Miss Ingham's day, and along with aromatherapy (see Chapter 7), has become one of the most favoured complementary therapies with nurses in the United Kingdom.

A 'treatment' (although practitioners might prefer not to use a word with such resonances of therapeutics) with some resemblance to reflexology is the *metamorphic technique*, which first appeared in the late 1960s, being developed by a naturopath and reflexologist, Robert St John. This is based on the idea that the foot mirrors the nine months of gestation; mental, physical, emotional and spiritual patterns, set before birth, can be felt in altered states of the foot's surfaces. With a feathery touch, the practitioner seeks to 'smooth out' these areas, thus subtly altering the states that led to ill health or stress. In a paper which outlines twenty-six ways in which metamorphic technique and reflexology differ, Gonzalez and Saint-Pierre state that metamorphic technique seeks not to treat particular ailments, but instead 'provides an environment within which the energy of the symptoms can move in a way that is right'; illness is seen as 'manifestations of energy'. There is not space within this book to do the subject justice; interested readers should start with Gonzales and Saint-Pierre's paper, 'Any difference between reflexology and the metamorphic technique?' (see 'Further reading', below).

Another technique which might be mentioned briefly is *VacuFlex reflexology*, which combines reflexology, 'cupping' (the use of vacuums on the skin surface), and acupressure (see shiatsu, Chapter 4, and acupuncture, Chapter 13). In this treatment, 'boots', connected to a vacuum pump, are put on the feet; when the pump is activated, the reflexes are stimulated. Treatment is then guided along lines of traditional Chinese medicine. Some reflexologists, however, would say that any technique employing tools of any kind is not, strictly speaking, reflexology, which they believe to be 'hands only'.

Details on how to obtain further information on metamorphosis and VacuFlex can be found under 'Resources', below.

Further reading

- Bayly, D. E. 1982. *Reflexology Today*, revd edn. Wellingborough: Thorsons.
- Dougans, I. & S. Ellis 1992. *The Art of Reflexology*. Shaftesbury: Element.
- Gonzales, M.-A. & G. Saint-Pierre 1992. Any difference between reflexology and the metamorphic technique? *Metamorphosis* **26**: 69–71.
- Grant, B. 1993. *A–Z of Natural Healthcare*. London: Macdonald Optima.

What is reflexology?

Reflexology involves the application of pressure to one part of the body – usually, but by no means always, the feet – to produce effects in other parts of the body.

The growth of interest in recent years among nurses has been phenomenal, and the pages of nursing journals contain a bewildering array of advertisements for establishments offering training in the technique.

The theory underlying reflexology is that the body is divided into ten **longitudinal zones**, with five closely associated zones on each arm (Figure 5.1), within which all the structures are connected by a flow of energy. The five areas on each foot and hand are, of course, part of the five zones on each side of the body: applying pressure on a **reflex point** within any one area will thus have corresponding effects on different organs lying within that zone (Figure 5.2). The application of local pressure also stimulates blood supply to the area.

The resemblance between this theory and that of traditional Chinese medicine, which postulates a flow of energy along Meridians (see Chapters 4 and 14), is striking, and at least one reflexologist has suggested that the concepts are identical (Dougans & Ellis 1992).

In addition to the longitudinal zones, there are **transverse zones** (Figure 5.3), which enable practitioners to draw up a kind of grid system for the identification of reflex points; and finally, there are **cross-reflexes** in which a relationship exists between different points on each side of the body. If, for any reason, pressure cannot be applied to the relevant reflex (for example, following soft-tissue injury), the cross-reflexes provide an alternative.

Crystalline deposits are said to build up in the reflexes of the feet, causing problems with related organs, and leading to ill-health; opinion is divided as to whether they are caused by disturbances in the energy flow, or are causative in themselves. The

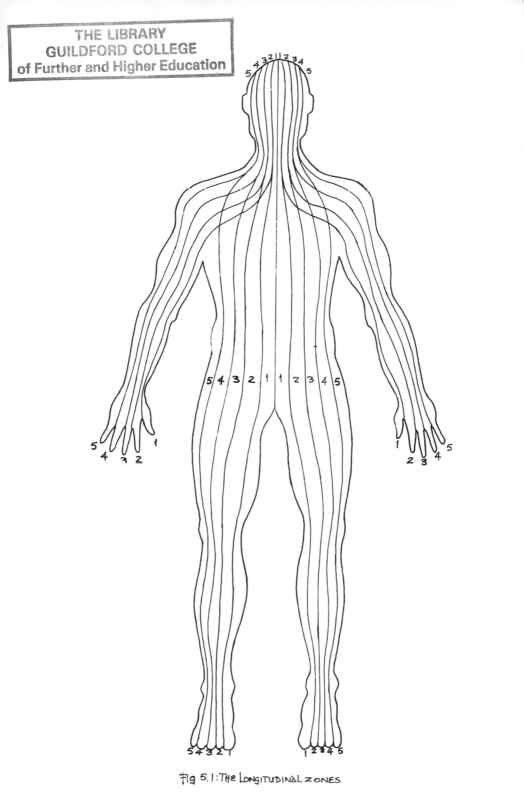

Fig 5.1: The Longitudinal zones

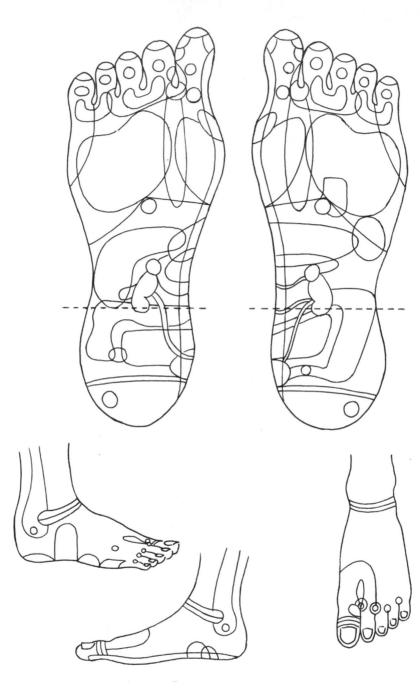

Fig 5.2 : Reflex points of the feet

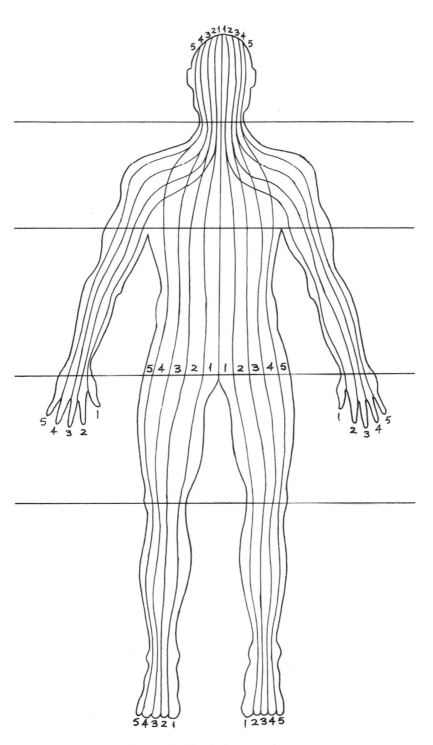

Fig 5.3: THE TRANSVERSE ZONES

reflexologist may use the presence of these deposits to 'read' the feet, and treatment consists of breaking them down with firm but gentle compression.

Several authors have attempted to explain reflexology's mode of action in the light of current knowledge about neurology. For some time, it has been known that there are areas on the surface of the body which seem to 'represent' internal organs; the nerve supplies are related, either directly or indirectly, because their embryological development was close. The best known of these associations is probably that seen in angina pectoris, where the first sign of oxygen deprivation to heart muscle is manifested as tingling or pain in the left arm; another is shoulder-tip pain, which can be the result of an ectopic pregnancy (in which the fertilised egg fails to reach the uterus, and develops in the Fallopian tube) or an abscess under the diaphragm. It has been considered possible that stimulation to the body's surface can, in some cases, directly affect the functioning of internal organs, but further evidence is needed to establish whether such connections exist between the feet and all other parts of the body.

The theory behind reflexology as a therapy can perhaps best be summed up as an attempt to restore the body's natural balance by the correction of problems of circulation – of blood, lymph, and of an intangible energy flow – thereby encouraging the clearance of toxins, and so allowing the body to heal itself (Norman & Cowan 1989). In addition, the importance of physical contact cannot be overstressed, and the relaxing effects of the treatment allow many people to open up and talk freely about their problems, which may be a therapy to itself.

An interesting debate seems to exist among practitioners as to what, exactly, the word 'reflexology' refers to. Some texts say that a 'reflex' is an involuntary response to a stimulus, and it describes the effect of pressure, applied to the hands or feet, on distant organs; but most say that the word is derived from the 'reflection' of physiological systems on the sole of the feet, and do not give any other interpretation.

Visiting a reflexologist

As with most of the other therapies described in this book, a large part of the first session will be devoted to collecting information about past and present health, and possibly finding out something about the person's lifestyle.

Treatment consists of the person sitting in a comfortable position, with the legs raised, while the practitioner first examines the feet. Pressure is then applied to all areas on both feet, using the thumbs and fingers. The 'feel' of certain areas, which may be particularly tender, indicate to the reflexologist which areas are deserving of special attention.

According to therapists, it is unusual for anyone not to be able to tolerate this procedure, however sensitive or ticklish their feet may be (Gore 1990).

A treatment can take up to 45 minutes, after which the person should feel more relaxed. The number of treatment sessions required will vary greatly from individual to individual, with some practitioners recommending an interval of at least a week between sessions, while others might feel that gentle daily sessions are appropriate.

As the body's natural healing processes assert themselves, transient effects may be noted. Old health problems, which were not fully resolved, may flare up again temporarily, but this is seen as a positive sign. There may be increased excretory activity, with the kidneys and digestive tract appearing to have speeded up, while a runny nose or ticklish cough may be a problem for a short while. Again, these are interpreted as positive signs that the body is working harder to clear toxins from the system. These signs are not seen in everyone, though.

An important point which should be made here is that reflexologists do not 'diagnose', according to the codes of practice of the major organisations; they can identify problems, but it is not within their remit to append names to them, as a medical practitioner would.

Indications

While reflexology does not really appear to have a role in the treatment of most acute conditions – although many practitioners would disagree – it may have some value as a complement to more 'orthodox' therapies.

Standard texts list over a hundred medical conditions which practitioners believe can be helped by reflexology, in addition to its use as a prognostic aid, in identifying potential problems, and as a relaxation technique. Among these are skin problems such as acne, some allergic responses, eczema, and psoriasis; disorders of the gastro-intestinal tract, including heartburn, constipation, and diarrhoea; problems which may be exacerbated by stress (for example, asthma and migraines); menstrual problems; and pain, particularly in sciatica and arthritis.

People with progressive disorders, such as multiple sclerosis, may find that their control of muscle function, both skeletal and in the bladder and bowel, is improved by reflexology, according to practitioners.

The area of infertility is one that some practitioners say could find reflexology useful, success having been claimed with raising low sperm counts, and low ovulation rates (Martin 1993); at the time of writing, however, this has not been documented.

A more complete list can be found in the texts listed under 'Recommended reading'.

Many of reflexology's claimed benefits may in fact come from its use as a stress-relieving therapy, which can prevent many health problems from appearing in the first place.

Contra-indications

When there are circulatory disorders of the lower limb, such as deep vein thrombosis, leg ulcers or phlebitis, caution must be exercised; only very experienced reflexologists are likely to have the necessary skills to avoid exacerbating the problem.

Reflexology can help relieve some problems associated with pregnancy, according to practitioners, but again caution must be exercised; most therapists would not treat a pregnant woman without her doctor's consent, and would be unhappy with the idea of a student carrying out such treatment.

A person who is psychotic, or taking large doses of psychoactive drugs, would be unlikely to benefit from reflexology.

If renal calculi are suspected, the renal reflexes are avoided; similarly, if the patient has large gallstones, the gallbladder and liver reflexes are not touched. This, according to reflexologists, is because the stones may move as a result.

Patients with pacemakers should get permission from their doctor to have reflexology, or the chest area on the left foot should be avoided as it has been known for the pacemaker to move after treatment (Martin 1993).

Research

Although there are a number of descriptions of how individual health-care professionals have successfully introduced reflexology into their areas of work, and almost all texts on the subject include detailed case histories (see 'Recommended reading'), it is extremely difficult to find details of any clinical trials. A literature search carried out by the Royal College of Nursing Library failed to discover any such research, and the British Library's section which deals with complementary therapies did not know of anything in this area.

Some practitioners say that as the therapy is so closely tailored to the needs of individuals, few research techniques, if any, can be applied to the study of reflexology. Another common complaint seems to be that medical staff are unwilling to help in such studies – possibly because they believe it to be an 'untested' therapy ... a belief backed by the lack of research evidence.

As the therapy becomes more widely known, it is hoped that some ingenious reflexologist will find a way around these problems; in the meantime, some co-operation from the medical profession might do much to speed the process.

Implications for nursing

Along with several other therapies discussed elsewhere in this book, reflexology is of particular interest to nurses: the basics can be learned in a relatively small number of lessons, avoiding some of the problems encountered in applying for study leave; it is a relatively safe procedure, with few contra-indications (although where caution is called for, the results of ignoring it can be serious); it requires no special tools or equipment; patients or clients tend to enjoy the procedure; and, most importantly, it seems to have beneficial effects, judging by the occasional reports seen in the nursing press. In addition, it is possible for individuals to practise some reflexology on themselves, which is helpful for anyone wishing to make up their own mind about possible benefits and drawbacks. However, no reputable school will award a certificate until a lengthy theoretical and practical course has been completed (see 'Resources').

Although the foundations of reflexology were laid down some time ago, it is still a 'new' therapy, in comparison with some of the other treatments being used by nurses, midwives and health visitors today. In a few years' time, when more nurses have had time to evaluate their experiences of using reflexology in their place of work, it may be possible to give a more complete assessment.

Examples of the use of reflexology in nursing and health care

In postnatal care

A nurse working in Wales has described using the therapy on a postnatal ward, where she felt it proved to be of use to both mothers and babies.

- Evans, M. 1990. Reflex zone therapy for mothers. *Nursing Times* 86(4): 29–31.

Suzanne Adamson is a health visitor in London who runs courses on massage and reflexology for new mothers, and believes that in the three years it has been running, many of those mothers' children have enjoyed better health than might otherwise have been the case.

– Sofroniou, P. 1993. Reflexology: the practitioner's story. In Booth, B.: *Complementary Therapy*. London: NT/Macmillan.

In cancer care

In an integrated model of care for cancer patients, devised jointly by the Bristol Cancer Help Centre and the oncology department of Hammersmith Hospital, London, reflexology is seen as an important adjunct to that care, and nurses are encouraged to undergo training.

– Burke, C. & K. Sikora, 1992. Cancer – the dual approach. *Nursing Times* **88**(38): 62–6.

Therapies that use touch

The therapeutic value of complementary therapies using touch – including reflexology – was looked at by a nurse as part of a degree in nursing studies, and she has written about trying to integrate her findings into day-to-day practice.

– Smith, M. 1990. Healing through touch. *Nursing Times* **86**(4): 31–2.

A pioneering course

Reflexology is one of the therapies included in a pioneering course on complementary therapies for nurses, run at St George's and Roehampton College of Health Studies, London.

– Mantle, F. 1992. Complementary care. *Nursing Times* **88**(18): 44–5.

Resources

Training and regulation

There is some variation in the time needed to complete a course in reflexology, depending on the establishment offering it. Jane Foulkes (1991) points out that course providers make different assumptions about prospective students' level of prior knowledge, which obviously affect the projected time to completion; someone with little knowledge of biology, for example, could be at a distinct disadvantage if he or she were to undertake the same course as a trained nurse.

Mary Martin, founder of the Association of Reflexologists, believes that poorly-trained therapists have harmed the therapy's standing. The course at her own school requires a minimum of 300 hours' theoretical study and practical work in a nine-month, part-time course, the clinical element including giving 60 treatments in a six-month period. The final written and practical examinations are assessed externally.

Reflexology does not currently have a single professional body to which all practitioners can apply for membership, but two main ones are the Association of Reflexologists and the British Reflexology Association.

Association of Reflexologists (AR)
27 Old Gloucester Street, London WC1 3XX.

The Association is not affiliated to any one school, but full membership is only open to reflexologists who have trained on a course accredited by the Association, holding a 'recognised certificate or diploma', who have been in practice for a year, and who agree to be bound by the Association's rules and ethical code. Full members may call themselves 'Registered Reflexologist', and use the letters MAR after their names.

There is a Practitioner Referral Register of qualified members, which the public may consult.

Details of the Register, the Association's continuing education programme, standards in education, training establishments offering accredited courses, and its quarterly journal *Reflexions*, are available from the above address on request.

British Reflexology Association (BRA)
Monks Orchard, Whitbourne, Worcester WR6 5RB.

The BRA was founded in 1985, and its official teaching body is the Bayly School of Reflexology in Worcester. It has a register of members, published annually and updated three times a year.

Graduates from the Bayly School may apply for membership after a minimum one year in practice; they may then use the title 'Registered Reflexologist', and append the letters MBRA to their name. Members have insurance cover. Anyone undergoing training at the Association's school can apply for student membership, with optional insurance.

Details of the Register, the Association newsletter *Footprints* and lecture days can be obtained from the Secretary.

Other useful addresses

Association of VacuFlex Reflexologists (AVR)
Further information can be obtained from: 1 Woodland Park, off Boxhill Road, Tadworth, Surrey KT20 7JL.

Metamorphic Association (MA)
67 Ritherdon Road, London SW17 8QE.

Recommended reading

- Bayly, D. E. 1982. *Reflexology Today*, revd edn. Wellingborough: Thorsons.
- Dougans, I. & S. Ellis 1992. *The Art of Reflexology: a step-by-step guide*. Shaftesbury: Element.
- Goodwin, H. 1988. Reflex zone therapy. In Rankin-Box, D. (ed.): *Complementary Health Therapies: a guide for nurses and the caring professions*. London: Chapman & Hall.
- Gore, A. 1990. *Reflexology*. London: Macdonald Optima.
- Hall, N. M. 1986. *Reflexology – a patient's guide*. Wellingborough: Thorsons.
- Norman, L. & T. Cowan 1989. *The Reflexology Handbook*. London: Piatkus.

References

- Bayly, D. E. 1982. *Reflexology Today*, revd edn. Wellingborough: Thorsons.
- Dougans, I. & S. Ellis 1992. *The Art of Reflexology: a step-by-step guide*. Shaftesbury: Element.
- Foulkes, J. 1991. *Complementary Therapies Career Handbook*. London: Headway.
- Gore, A. 1990. *Reflexology*. London: Macdonald Optima.
- Martin, M. 1993. Personal communication (June).
- Norman, L. & T. Cowan (1989). *The Reflexology Handbook*. London: Piatkus.

6 AROMATHERAPY

Historical background

Whose spirits are not lifted by the smell of fresh mint, tarragon or parsley in a salad, by a rose-scented pot-pourri in the living room, or by the heady aroma of jasmine and honeysuckle in a summer garden? We know almost instinctively that plants and their aromas are in some way beneficial, and since humankind's earliest history we have incorporated them into our religions, medicine, cooking and beauty preparations.

Archaeologists have found evidence that, as far back as 3000 BC, the people of the Indus Valley civilisation (in present-day Pakistan) knew how to distil oils. But the use of aromatic plants and oils probably dates back to the first time someone threw a piece of wood on the fire and liked the smell it gave to the smoke. From a simple act such as this, our predecessors must have gone on to experiment with the properties of different plants and then put them to use.

Many ancient cultures used aromatics; of these, the Egyptians are probably the best known. They, too, had been using them since 3000 BC for perfumes, in embalming practices and in their medicines. The Ancient Greeks then built on this knowledge, adding uses of their own; they used olive oil, for example, to absorb the aroma of plants. As the Romans employed Greek physicians, the use of aromatics spread still further. The Arabs in turn made translations of the Graeco-Roman medical texts and went on to take medicine in general to new heights. One of the most famous Arab doctors was Abu Ali Ibn Sina (AD 980–1037), or Avicenna as he was known in the West. He described over eight hundred plants and their effects on the human body, as well as developing a method of distilling essential oils. Further East, in India and China, there are also writings, dating from 2000 BC, which describe the use of aromatics for religious and medical purposes.

In Europe, the use of herbs and plants was well established from the earliest times. During mediaeval times, for example, floors were strewn with strong-smelling herbs to cover the general stench and to repel many disease-carrying insects; herbal posies were carried to ward off the plague, and lavender bags were placed in cupboards to protect linen from moths. In the same period, aromatic oils from the East were brought to Europe by traders and by the Crusaders, who returned from their holy wars with the knowledge of how to distil them.

During the Rennaissance, the distillation process was industrialised: thus began the chemical investigation of essential oils. By the 19th century, chemists were beginning to identify the actual constituents of plant oils; this led to the development of synthetic counterparts, and contributed to the growth of the pharmaceutical industry.

Aromatherapy as practised today (the therapeutic use of specially-prepared plant essential oils) is a relatively new discipline. It was a French chemist called René-Maurice Gattefosse who, in 1928, first used the term. His family owned a perfume business, and while working in his laboratory one day, he burnt his hand. Noticing some neat lavender oil nearby, he plunged his hand into the container. To his surprise the burns healed within hours, leaving no scars. As a result, he went on to investigate other oils and to use them in dermatological preparations. In his scientific writings on the subject, he always referred to 'aromatherapie', and the term stuck.

From the 1950s onwards, another Frenchman, Dr Jean Valnet, began using essential oils in his medical practice. His success prompted others to follow and stimulated research. In fact, his books are still considered classics today (see 'Resources').

In the UK, the popularity of aromatherapy is more recent – although aromatherapist Marguerite Maury was using essential oils in the 1960s – and it is probably more widely known here as a type of beauty treatment than as a therapy.

Further reading

- Gattefosse, M. 1992. René-Maurice Gattefosse – the father of modern aromatherapy. *The International Journal of Aromatherapy* (Winter 1992), 4(4): 18–19.
- Lawless, J. 1992. *The Encyclopaedia of Essential Oils.* Shaftesbury: Element.
- Valnet, J. 1992. *The Practice of Aromatherapy.* Saffron Walden: C. W. Daniel.
- Worwood, V. 1992. *The Fragrant Pharmacy.* London: Bantam.

What is aromatherapy?

Aromatherapy refers to the therapeutic use of specially-prepared **essential** or **aromatic oils**. The oils can be found in different parts of plants including the flowers, leaves, seeds, wood, roots, and bark.

Each oil comprises various constituents. The main ones are **hydrocarbons** called *terpenes,* and **oxygenated compounds** which include *esters, aldehydes, ketones, alcohols, phenols* and *oxides. Lactones, sulphur* and *nitrogen* compounds can also be found in some oils.

Chemists have found that essential oils interact with our bodies in three ways:

- *pharmacologically,* through chemical changes when oils enter the bloodstream and react with hormones, enzymes, and so on;
- *physiologically,* by producing an effect on the body, such as sedation or stimulation; and
- *psychologically,* when the aroma of an oil is inhaled and we react to the smell.

All oils are readily absorbed through the skin.

Using essential oils

According to aromatherapists, there are many different ways in which essential oils can be applied. One of the skills of an aromatherapist is – they will tell you – to select the most appropriate oil or oils for each client.

Massage

Massage is the most common way of applying essential oils. Usually a full body massage is given; this in itself can be very relaxing and beneficial (see Chapter 3).

An aromatherapist will select the appropriate oils for the client and blend them with a **base oil**. Any light vegetable, nut or seed oil can be used, but **almond oil** and **grapeseed oil** are particularly popular bases.

It is important that only small amounts of essential oils are used. Any oil can be harmful if not used sparingly. Unless a trained aromatherapist, a nurse should not use more than 3–5 drops of essential oil to 1 tablespoon of base oil. Some oils can irritate the skin (see 'Baths' below), so oils should be used with care.

Some oils make the skin more sensitive to ultraviolet light and should therefore not be applied before going out into strong sunlight or before using a sunbed. These oils include Angelica, Bergamot, Cumin, Lemon, Lime, Orange and Lemon Verbena. As a general rule, it is advisable not to use any essential oils before going into strong sunlight.

Skin oils and lotions

The same principles apply here as for massage, the only difference being that the essential oils are combined with a base oil and a richer oil such as Jojoba or Avocado, or in a simple cold cream. Some aromatherapists may add essential oils to an alcohol-based lotion in treating certain conditions.

Such oils and lotions are used for treating the skin. They are applied with gentle circular motions to ensure the skin is not pulled unnecessarily.

Baths

No more than 5–8 drops of essential oil should be added to a bath, and this should be done once the bath is full and the temperature adjusted.

It is important to be especially careful in the use of oils which may be irritating to the skin. Such oils should be diluted in a base oil (3–4 drops per tablespoon of base should be added to the base oil). Oils which may irritate the skin include Basil, Lemon, Lemongrass, Lemon Verbena, Melissa, Peppermint, Thyme, Cinnamon Leaf, Sweet Fennel, Siberian Fir Needle, Parsley Seed, and Pimenta Leaf. None of these oils should be used with people who have skin or allergy problems.

Douches

For a douche, 5–10 drops of essential oil should be added for every litre of warm water used.

Hot and cold compresses

Compresses are used to relieve pain or to reduce inflammation and swelling. No more than 4 or 5 drops of essential oil should be added to a bowl of hot or ice-cold (as appropriate) water. A clean cotton cloth or cotton wool can then be dipped into the solution, excess water squeezed out, and the resultant compress placed on the affected area. Compresses should be replaced as necessary.

Neat application

Undiluted essential oils should never be applied to the skin, with the exceptions of Lavender oil for burns, insect bites, and cuts; Lemon oil for warts; and Tea Tree for spots and fungal infections.

Internal use

The International Federation of Aromatherapists (see 'Resources') advises that essential oils should *not* be taken internally. Some aromatherapists disagree, but it is certainly the case that untrained individuals should never take or give essential oils internally.

Flower waters

To make **flower waters**, add 20–30 drops of essential oil to 100 ml of spring water. The mixture should then be left in the dark for a few days, after which it should be filtered through coffee filter paper. Such flower waters are used in skin treatments.

Vaporisation

Essential oils can be added to special burners to freshen a room or alter the mood. Burners must be put in a safe place, particularly if there are children around.

A new device, called a LANDEL diffuser, has been developed for safe use in places such as hospitals. According to practitioners, it is very effective and is not a fire hazard. For more information, contact the distributors: 'Essentially Yours', PO Box 38, Romford, Essex.

Steam inhalation

For inhalation, 5 drops of oil can be added to a bowl of hot water. This can then be inhaled under a towel.

A properly trained aromatherapist will use essential oils within a holistic framework, seeking to maintain a balance of mental, physical and spiritual health. As well as using essential oils, an aromatherapist will also look at diet, exercise and other elements of the client's lifestyle that may contribute to his or her health and well-being.

Provided that instructions are followed carefully, essential oils can usually be used safely by untrained individuals. There are simple remedies for minor ailments, first aid, relaxation, and cosmetics, all of which are said to be effective. However, anyone using essential oils should first check the contra-indications for each oil, and if unsure of how to proceed, should take advice from a trained aromatherapist. Just because something smells nice, this does not mean that it is harmless. Nurses without recognised training in aromatherapy should never use essential oils with patients.

Further reading

– Davis, P. 1988. *Aromatherapy: an A–Z*. Saffron Walden: C. W. Daniel.
– Genders, R. A. 1977. *A Book of Aromatics*. London: Darton, Longman & Todd.
– Price, S. 1985. *Practical Aromatherapy*. Wellingborough: Thorsons.
– Ryan, D. 1984. *The Aromatherapy Handbook*. London: Century.
– Tisserand, R. 1990. *Aromatherapy for Everyone*. London: Arkana.
– Worwood, V. 1992. *The Fragrant Pharmacy*. London: Bantam.

Indications

Aromatherapy claims to be a useful complement to many other natural therapies and to orthodox medicine. The International Federation of Aromatherapists, for example, says that aromatherapy 'enhances well-being, relieves stress and helps in the rejuvenation and regeneration of the human body'.

On the one hand it can usually be safely used by anyone, provided that instructions are followed carefully and contra-indications noted; and on the other, trained aromatherapists are treating a very wide range of illnesses and conditions. Some of the properties ascribed to essential oils are listed in Box 6.1.

BOX 6.1
COMMONLY USED ESSENTIAL OILS AND SOME PROPERTIES ASCRIBED TO THEM

Basil (*Ocimum basilicum*) Cephalic (clears the mind and stimulates mental activity); sudorific (promotes sweating); tonic.

Bergamot (*Citrus bergamia*) Analgesic; antidepressant; anti-inflammatory; antiseptic; bactericidal; bacteriostatic (inhibits the growth of bacteria); deodorant; expectorant; febrifugal (reduces fever); sedative; vulnerary (helps wounds to heal).

Camomile, Roman (*Anthemis nobilis*) Analgesic; antidepressant; anti-inflammatory; cholagogic (stimulates the flow of bile); diuretic; emmenagogic (encourages menstruation); febrifugal; hepatic (strengthens the liver); hypnotic (induces sleep); nervine (strengthens the nervous system); sudorific; tonic; vasoconstrictive; vulnerary.

Clary Sage (*Salvia sclarea*) Antidepressant; aphrodisiac; deodorant; emmenagogic; hypertensive; sedative; uterine (has a tonic action on the womb); vulnerary.

Cypress (*Cupressus sempervirens*) Astringent; deodorant; diuretic; hepatic.

Eucalyptus (*Eucalyptus globulus*) Antiseptic; bactericidal; bacteriostatic; deodorant; expectorant; febrifugal; rubefacient (produces warmth and redness when applied to the skin); stimulant (increases the activity of the body generally, or of a specific organ).

Garlic (*Allium sativum*) Antiviral; bactericidal; bacteriostatic; detoxicant; immunostimulant.

Geranium (*Pelargonium graveolens/Pelargonium roseum*) Antidepressant; diuretic; stimulant; tonic.

Jasmine (*Jasminum grandiflorum*) Antidepressant; aphrodisiac; uterine.

Juniper (*Juniperus communis*) Antiseptic; astringent; bactericidal; bacteriostatic; detoxicant; diuretic; emmenagogic; rubefacient; sedative; sudorific; tonic.

Lavender (*Lavandula angustifolia*) Analgesic; antidepressant; anti-inflammatory; antiseptic; antiviral; bactericidal; bacteriostatic; bechic (eases coughing); cholagogic; cytophylactic (a cell regenerator); deodorant; emmenagogic; fungicidal; hypnotic; hypotensive; immunostimulant; nervine; sedative; tonic; vulnerary.

Spanish Marjoram (*Thymus mastichina*) Anaphrodisiac (reduces sexual response); emmenagogic; expectorant; hypnotic; hypotensive; nervine; rubefacient; sedative; tonic; vasodilator.

Orange Blossom Flowers (*Neroli*) (*Citrus aurantium*) Antidepressant; aphrodisiac; cytophylactic; deodorant; hypnotic; sedative; tonic.

Peppermint (*Mentha piperita*) Cholagogic; febrifugal; hepatic; stimulant; sudorific.

Rose (*Rosa centifolia*) Antidepressant; aphrodisiac; astringent; detoxicant; emmenagogic; sedative; tonic; uterine; vasoconstrictive.

Rosemary (*Rosmarinus officinalis*) Analgesic; antiseptic; bactericidal; cephalic; cholagogic; diuretic; emmenagogic; hepatic; hypertensive; nervine; rubefacient; stimulant; sudorific.

Sandalwood (*Santalum album*) Antidepressant; antiseptic; aphrodisiac; astringent; bacteriostatic; bechic; diuretic; expectorant; sedative.

Tea Tree (*Melaleuca alternifolia*) Antiseptic; antiviral; bactericidal; bacteriostatic; cytophylactic; febrifugal; fungicidal; immunostimulant; sudorific; tonic; vulnerary.

Thyme (*Thymus vulgaris*) Antiseptic; bacteriostatic; bechic; hepatic.

Ylang-Ylang (*Canangium odoratum*) Antidepressant; aphrodisiac; hypnotic; hypotensive.

As essential oils are widely used in the fragrance and flavour industries, the properties of the oils have, in the main, been well researched and have been ascribed with care.

According to Robert Tisserand (1990) aromatherapists in the UK 'do not treat the more serious ailments such as nervous diseases (multiple sclerosis, Parkinsonism, epilepsy, etc.), cancers and serious infections such as hepatitis, diphtheria, meningitis, AIDS, venereal diseases and so on'. However, he claims that aromatherapy is 'of considerable help in the area of common, stress-related and other minor disorders for which the busy general practitioner often finds it difficult to provide a solution'. Examples of such conditions are pre-menstrual syndrome, moderate anxiety or depression, sleeping problems, minor aches and pains, migraines, digestive disorders, skin problems such as eczema and acne, and minor infections such as thrush and cystitis.

There is a wide range of books on aromatherapy (see 'Resources'), many of which offer simple remedies for personal use. A small selection of such remedies is reproduced in Box 6.2. None of these remedies should be used by a nurse with patients unless she or he has undergone recognised training in aromatherapy.

BOX 6.2
USING ESSENTIAL OILS AT HOME

Baths

Patricia Davis, in her book *Aromatherapy: an A–Z* (1988), recommends the following baths for relaxation and to promote sleep:

- Lavender: 4 drops
- Bergamot: 2 drops

or

- Lavender: 4 drops
- Marjoram: 2 drops

She also suggests the following baths to help with symptoms of colds, flu and other viral infections, particularly if they are used at the *onset* of a cold, etc:

- Lavender: 2 drops
- Bergamot: 2 drops
- Tea Tree: 2 drops
  (for evening use)

or

- Lavender: 2 drops
- Rosemary: 2 drops
- Tea Tree: 2 drops
  (for morning use)

- Lavender: 3 drops
- Thyme: 2 drops
- Tea Tree: 1 drop
  (if the throat is sore)

or

- Lavender: 2 drops
- Frankincense: 2 drops
- Niaouli: 2 drops
  (if there is a cough)

Hair preparations

Julia Lawless, in her book *The Encyclopaedia of Essential Oils* (1992), suggests using essential oils in hair preparations – for example, 4 or 5 drops of Rosemary or Camomile can be added to a mild shampoo to improve the general health of hair; or 4 or 5 drops of Bergamot or Tea Tree can be added to help with the problem of dandruff.

Contra-indications

Certain essential oils should never be used, except by a qualified aromatherapist, as they are known to be toxic or to cause serious skin irritation (see Box 6.3).

BOX 6.3
ESSENTIAL OILS THAT SHOULD NEVER BE USED IN A THERAPEUTIC CONTEXT

- Almond, Bitter
- Aniseed
- Boldo – *leaf*
- Calmus
- Camphor, Brown
- Camphor, Yellow
- Cassia
- Cinnamon – *bark*
- Clove – *bud*
- Clove – *leaf*
- Clove – *stem*
- Costus
- Elecampane
- Fennel, Bitter
- Horseradish
- Hyssop
- Jaborandi – *leaf*
- Mugwort (Armoise)
- Mustard
- Origanum
- Origanum, Spanish
- Pennyroyal, European
- Pennyroyal, North American
- Pine, Dwarf
- Rue
- Sage
- Sassafras
- Sassafras, Brazilian
- Savin
- Savory, Summer
- Savory, Winter
- Southernwood
- Tansy
- Thuja (Cedarleaf)
- Thuja Plicata
- Wintergreen
- Wormseed
- Wormwood

There are also oils which are contra-indicated for particular conditions. For example:

- Sweet Fennel and Rosemary should not be used if a person has *epilepsy*.
- Arnica, Basil, Clary Sage, Cypress, Juniper, Marjoram, Myrrh, Sage, and Thyme should not be used during *pregnancy*. Sweet Fennel and Rosemary should not be used in the first 3–4 months of *pregnancy*, and only well diluted in the later months. As Camomile and Lavender are described as emmenagogic, they should be used in small amounts by women who may be at risk of *miscarrying* or where there may be risk of any *abnormal bleeding*. Jasmine, Rose and Peppermint can be used in *pregnancy* in appropriate doses.

> - Rosemary, Sage and Thyme should not be used with anyone suffering from *high blood pressure.*
>
> Always check with a trained aromatherapist if the safety of using a particular oil is in doubt.
>
> For more information on the safety of oils, consult *The Essential Oils Safety Data Manual* (Saffron Walden: C. W. Daniel, 1988), compiled by Robert Tisserand of the Tisserand Institute (see 'Resources').

Research

For hundreds of years pharmacists and chemists have been analysing the therapeutic properties of essential oils. Much of the research has been undertaken in France and has not been translated into English. However, the International Federation of Aromatherapists, the Tisserand Institute, the International Society of Professional Aromatherapists, and the more recently formed Aromatherapy Organizations Council (see 'Resources') are all keen to promote research and do keep details of published research. Natural Therapies Database UK, formed in 1992, produces quarterly publications relating to aromatherapy research. For more information, write to 47 Ashby Avenue, Surrey KT9 2BT.

The range of research

The list of studies below is by no means comprehensive, but is intended to illustrate the range of research that has been undertaken to investigate the therapeutic effects of essential oils:

- Basset, I. B., D. L. Pannowitz & R. St C. Barneston, 1991. Tee Tree gel controls acne. *The International Journal of Aromatherapy* **3**(1): 14–15.
- Blackwell, R. 1991. An insight into aromatic oils: Lavender & Tea Tree. *British Journal of Phytotherapy* (Spring) **2**(1): 25–30.
- Bronough, R. L. 1990. *In vivo* percutaneous absorption of fragrance ingredients in rhesus monkeys and humans. *Food & Chemical Toxicology* **28** (part 5): 369–74.
- Deans, S. 1991. Plant volatile oils: the origins, composition and biological activities. *International Journal of Aromatherapy* **3**(1): 16.
- Ehlichman, H. 1991. Odor experience as an effective state: effects of odor pleasantness on cognition. Fragrance Research Fund: *Perfumier and Flavourist* (March 16): 11–12.
- King, J. 1983. Have the scents to relax. *World Medicine* (October) **1**: 29.
- Koedam, A. 1982. *Antimicrobial Activity of Essential Oils*. Stuttgart: Atherische Ole.
- Maibach, H. 1982. Cosmetic reactions. *Journal of the American Academy of Dermatology* **6**: 909–17.

- Mishra, A. K., *et al.* 1991. Fungistatic properties of essential oil of *Cinnamomum camphora*. *International Journal of Pharmacognosy* **29**(4): 2599–602.
- Rudzki, E. 1976. Essential oils: sensitivity to 35 oils. *Contributions in Dermatology* **2**: 196–200.
- Shumunes, E. 1984. Contact dermatitis in atopic people. *Dermatologic Clinics* **2**: 561–4.

An argument against massage with essential oils

An interesting paper which looks at what is known about the biological effects of essential oils and argues that aromatherapy should not include the application of essential oils by massage is to be found in *The International Journal of Aromatherapy*:

- Buchbauer, G. 1993. Molecular interaction: biological effects and modes of action of essential oils. *The International Journal of Aromatherapy* (Spring), 5(1): 11–14.

Nurse-led evaluations of aromatherapy

Evaluations of aromatherapy as a therapy are, unfortunately, much thinner on the ground. Most combine the use of a particular essential oil with massage. Nurses have been undertaking some research in this area, but it is generally very small-scale, involving only a handful of patients. Potentially, nurses are in a position to produce excellent research in this area, but until more nurses become properly trained, the research will remain of limited value. Three small-scale studies by nurses are listed below.

Reduction of pain

Massage with Lavender oil in an almond-oil base was shown to reduce self-assessed pain levels in 50 per cent of the patients receiving it.

- Wollfson, A. & D. Hewitt, 1992. Intensive aromacare. *International Journal of Aromatherapy* 4(2): 12–14.

Benefits of foot massage

A study by Dawn Hewitt, a staff nurse at the Royal Sussex Hospital in Brighton, suggests that giving patients in intensive-care and coronary-care units a twenty-minute foot massage with Lavender oil could reduce heart rate, respiratory rate, blood pressure, pain, and wakefulness. The reductions were more more marked in patients who received the massage with the essential oil than with patients who received massage alone, or patients who had an undisturbed rest of twenty minutes.

– Nursing Times 1992. Massage with Lavender oil lowered tension. *Nursing Times* **88**(25): 8.

Reduction of stress

In a randomised double-blind trial, two Lavender oils (*Lavandula burnatii* and *Lavandula angustifolia*) were topically applied on post-cardiotomy patients. The emotional- and behavioural-stress levels of 28 patients were evaluated pre- and post-treatment, on two consecutive days. The therapeutic effects of the two lavender oils appeared different: *L. burnatii* was almost twice as effective as *L. angustifolia*. The results lend support to the supposition that aromatherapy does have a therapeutic effect that is not simply due to massage, touch or placebo, and that the selection of the most appropriate oils is indeed important.

– Buckle, J. 1993. Aromatherapy: does it matter which Lavender essential oil is used? *Nursing Times* **89**(20): 32–5.

Endometriosis trial

The International Federation of Aromatherapists has undertaken a study of the use of aromatherapy for stress and pain reduction in the treatment of endometriosis patients. According to Valerie Worwood, chairman of research for the Federation, the study was conducted over 24 weeks, initially using 25 aromatherapists who were full members of the IFA. All volunteer patients were members of the British Endometriosis Society, and had the consent of their gynaecologists or GPs to participate. All therapists were required to attend an information day at which all known aspects of the disease were discussed, including conventional treatment and how aromatherapy could be included as part of the care. The patients came to discuss their individual problems and conditions, which gave the therapists an insight into the psychological aspects and the disruption to the patients' lifestyles. The therapists were taught the specialised techniques needed for patient care, and a back-up hotline was provided.

'At the conclusion, all who had participated were genuinely pleased they had volunteered. Patients wrote letters of thanks, some sent flowers, and there were two pregnancies. Our preliminary findings show us that aromatherapy has a place in the care and treatment of endometriosis, that the majority of patients experienced less stress and tension and felt able to cope better with the condition, and had less pain. Regulation of the cycle and overall health improvements were also found', says Ms Worwood. For more details, contact the IFA.

– Personal communication 1993.

Care of rheumatoid arthritis

A further study looking at how aromatherapy can help in the improvement of lifestyle for people with rheumatoid arthritis is now underway. For further details, contact the IFA.

Implications for nursing

Aromatherapy is immensely popular with nurses, midwives and health visitors. It is already being used in a wide variety of settings (see below). Its popularity stems from the ease with which nurses perceive that it can be incorporated within their practice, and the positive feedback they receive from patients. A little Lavender oil on the pillow of a patient who cannot sleep, so the argument goes, can act as a simple, harmless sedative (Wise 1989); Rose Geranium has been used to help calm patients before an operation; and the use of Peppermint oil helped one group of patients accept their colostomies (MacKenzie & Gallacher 1989).

It is important, however, that nurses using essential oils do so in an informed way, and that they have undertaken a recognised course of study. Many oils are dangerous and the use of others is contra-indicated with some conditions. Unfortunately, there are nurse tutors 'teaching' aromatherapy to students after only a short course in the subject themselves, and often with no experience of aromatherapy as a practitioner.

It is also true that the right oils must be used. For example, only one of the four species of Lavender has a known sedative effect (*Lavandula angustifolia*), and the Lavender oil available in most pharmacies is apparently not made from this species (Buckle 1992).

The introduction of aromatherapy into a ward, unit or clinic should always be evaluated. That patients say they like it is good news, but nursing practice should be research-based. Findings from well-designed nursing research into aromatherapy could also help aromatherapy gain wider acceptance – particularly within the health service. 'Testing' an oil on a handful of patients in a 'pilot study'; however, does not constitute good research. Many trained aromatherapists are concerned at the ill-informed way in which some nurses are introducing aromatherapy into their practice. There is a real danger that as a result of essential oils being used in an uninformed way by nurses, a patient will be harmed and aromatherapy brought into disrepute.

For nurses who do not want to use aromatherapy themselves, but who wish to offer its benefits to their patients, the International Federation of Aromatherapists has, since 1988, been running the 'Aromatherapy In-Care Project'. This is a voluntary service whereby aromatherapists work alongside health professionals within the NHS. Hospices, intensive-care units, care of the elderly units and oncology units throughout the UK are participating in the project.

Certainly health professionals who have worked with aromatherapists as part of the project seem extremely pleased with the results. For example, one sister in charge of a hospice told the IFA, 'Aromatherapy often initiates conversation and the patients will sometimes talk of matters causing them great distress but which they have not felt free to voice before. The massage with relevant oils certainly helps to relieve pain and discomfort and is of tremendous value as an adjunct to medication.' And a Macmillan nurse reported that a young woman suffering from cancer found the aromatherapy sessions very relaxing. 'Her pain lessened and she says that following her treatment she was able to straighten out her legs for the first time in many months' (personal communication 1993).

Sadly the project has never been evaluated, and the IFA has lost a valuable opportunity to provide some useful research findings in favour of aromatherapy. For more information, contact the Coordinator of the Aromatherapy In-Care Project, c/o Department of Continuing Education, The Royal Masonic Hospital, Ravenscourt Park, London W6 0TN.

In 1993, the National Association of Health Authorities and Trusts published the findings of a national survey which examined purchasers' attitudes towards the availability of complementary therapies in the NHS (NAHAT 1993). More than 70 per cent of family health service authorities (FHSAs) and GP fundholders (GPFHs), and 65 per cent of district health authorities (DHAs), indicated that they were in favour of some or all complementary therapies being available on the NHS, free at the point of contact. About 20 per cent of DHAs thought aromatherapy should be available, as did just under 15 per cent of FHSAs and about 5 per cent of GPFHs. Two health-promotion clinics offering aromatherapy have been approved by FHSAs. DHAs had 17 contracts for aromatherapy which were part of a mainstream specialty contact, 3 which were separate contracts, and 2 with the private sector.

Aromatherapy was also mentioned as being used in radiotherapy, oncology/palliative care services, care of the elderly, and with people suffering from HIV/AIDS.

Examples of the use of aromatherapy in nursing and health care

In health visiting

Favre Armstrong, a health visitor working in Bath, is also a qualified aromatherapist. She regularly uses aromatherapy in her health-visiting practice. She has found aromatherapy helpful for a wide variety of conditions including arthritis, rheumatism, backache, sinusitis and catarrh, postnatal depression, menstrual problems, anxiety, and depression. She has also found that hypertensive patients feel the benefit of aromatherapy – their blood pressure usually drops several points during treatment.

– Armstrong, F. 1991. Scenting relief. *Nursing Times* **87**(10): 52–4.

In the care of the elderly

Sister Helen Passant has introduced a wide range of complementary therapies onto her ward. For example, she massaged patients with a mixture of Comfrey oil, Lavender oil and a carrier oil. She noticed a significant change in her patients: they needed less medication, they felt less pain, and they needed less sedation.

– Passant, H. 1990. A holistic approach to the ward. *Nursing Times* **86**(4): 26–8.

Registered mental nurse Mark Hardy, who works at the Old Manor Hospital in Salisbury, found that a natural and refreshing night's sleep can be obtained for elderly mentally-ill patients who have experienced difficulty in sleeping, without recourse to drugs. Lavender oil was diffused into the dormitory through a special air freshener.

– Hardy, M. 1991. Sweet-scented dreams. *The International Journal of Aromatherapy* **3**(1): 12–13.

In intensive care

Caroline Stevensen is a sister in an ITU unit at the Middlesex Hospital, London. She is also a qualified shiatsu practitioner, iridologist and aromatherapist. She has found that foot massage with Neroli essential oil contributed to a marked reduction in anxiety levels among patients who had undergone cardiac surgery.

– Stevensen, C. 1992. Measuring the effect of aromatherapy. *Nursing Times* **88**(41): 62–3.

In the treatment of people with epilepsy

At the Department of Psychiatry at the Queen Elizabeth Hospital in Birmingham, nurse Sarah Boden and colleagues Teena Clouston and Tim Betts have been using aromatherapy to treat ten patients with epilepsy. The treatment has produced a significant reduction in seizure frequency. Patients selected the oil to be used from a range of anticonvulsant to anxiolytic essential oils. The patients then had about six aromatherapy massages at weekly intervals with the chosen oil. Towards the end of the course a light hypnotic suggestion was used to help the patients develop the same relaxation response whenever they smelt the oil; thereafter they carried a small bottle of the oil with them, to inhale from if they were feeling tense or felt a seizure coming on.

– Personal communication 1993.

Resources

Buying and storing essential oils

Essential oils vary enormously in price and quality. It is important that any oil you buy is pure and not blended. A pure oil is one that has not been adulterated with chemicals or synthethic compounds and than comes from a named botanical plant from a definite geographical area.

Some oils are marketed as 'aromatherapy oils'. These are mixtures of an essential oil and a carrier oil. The proportion of essential oil in such products varies, and may be as little as 4 per cent.

Many aromatherapists recommend essential oils distilled from organically grown plants. Such oils should be grown according to strict guidelines such as those set down by the International Federation of Agricultural Organic Movements. The problem for the consumer is establishing whether oils marketed as organic are indeed so.

Natural Oils Research Association (NORA)
PO Box 1604, Windsor, Berkshire SL4 3YR.

This Association was set up to conduct educational courses and co-ordinate research into aromatics, essential oils, aromatherapy and phytotherapy. In 1990 it initiated the 'Aromark' programme to test and certificate oils.

Tisserand Institute
65 Church Road, Hove, East Sussex BN3 2BD (Tel. 0273 206640).

This is a training institute, set up in 1987; it also offers a consumer helpline (*Tel.* 0273 412139).

The Aromatherapy Organisations Council (see below) now has a trade section which oversees the sale of essential oils. However, it is worth asking aromatherapists where they get their oils, as a personal recommendation from a professional may be your only marker in what is still largely an unregulated market.

Storage

Oils should be stored in tightly closed bottles in a cool cupboard away from heat. Some oils, such as Jasmine and Neroli, should be kept in the fridge. The therapeutic effects of most oils will last for two or three years, except for citrus oils which last for one year only.

Training and regulation

As with many complementary therapies, there is no one organisation that can truly say it represents all aromatherapists in the UK. It is true to say, however, that efforts are being made to standardise and improve training programmes, and to ensure that all practising aromatherapists work within a recognised code of conduct and are properly insured.

The annotated list below gives details of some of the major aromatherapy organisations.

Aromatherapy Organisations Council (AOC)
3 Latymer Close, Braybrooke, Market Harborough, Leicester LE16 8LN.

According to Sylvia Baker, secretary to AOC, 'it is definitely the governing body unifying the various professional associations and training bodies'. It was set up in 1991 under the auspices of the umbrella organisation, the British Complementary Medicine Association (see Chapter 1), which acts as the facilitating body. In 1993 AOC represented 9 associations and 18 schools. A further 32 schools are represented indirectly through the associations. A list of members is available from the above address.

The aims and objectives of the AOC are as follows:

- to unify the profession by bringing together its various organisations;
- to establish common standards of training, and to ensure that all organisations registered with the Council provide appropriate standards of professional practice and conduct for their members;
- to act as a public watchdog;
- to provide for all organisations within aromatherapy a collective voice through which to initiate and sustain political dialogue with government, civil and medical bodies, in order to enhance the best interests of professional aromatherapy;
- to offer a mediation and arbitration service in any dispute involving aromatherapy organisations.

The AOC is not, however, a statutory governing body with legislative backing.

The AOC is active in the arena of training, and in 1992 announced that a minimum training standard of 180 class hours for students of aromatherapy had been set by the Council. This means, says the Council, that many schools have to upgrade their current training courses. It is also discussing progressive levels of training and is involved in consultations with the National Council for Vocational Qualifications.

International Federation of Aromatherapists (IFA)
C/o Department of Continuing Education, The Royal Masonic Hospital, Ravenscourt Park, London W6 0TN.

The IFA was formed in 1985 and is the oldest aromatherapy organisation. It has charitable status and more than 1300 members. The letters MIFA after a practitioner's name denote his or her membership of the IFA, and therefore that he or she has trained to a standard set by the IFA. A list of practitioners and accredited training schools is available from the IFA on receipt of a cheque for £1.10. The IFA has a code of practice backed up by disciplinary procedures, and claims to act on complaints; members can be struck off the practitioner list. The IFA also provides insurance for members.

The IFA is, it says, active in setting standards and in undertaking research (see 'Research' section). A spokeswoman for the IFA claims that they are 'the only independent representative body in the UK co-ordinating and encouraging the practice of aromatherapy', and the IFA has now withdrawn its membership of the AOC.

The IFA has set up a body to control training schools, and students must also sit IFA exams in addition to the schools exams. The IFA is, it says, 'active in putting syllabuses together'.

International Society of Professional Aromatherapists (ISPA)
41 Leicester Road, Hinckley, Leicester LE10 1LW.

The ISPA was set up in 1990 and in 1993 had 1361 members. It is a member of the AOC, and has an enforceable code of practice and ethics, insurance for members, and a register of members (available from the above address). It is keen to encourage research and to publish findings in its journal. The ISPA is also committed to improving standards, and validates training courses. The conditions of membership are strict, for example expecting members to engage in appropriate postgraduate studies each year in order to keep abreast of new knowledge and developments and to acquire new skills (minimum two days); not to attempt to treat conditions beyond their level of skill, but rather to refer them either to a more experienced colleague or the client's GP; and to seek to make and maintain professional relationships with the client's GP whenever possible, seeking his or her support and approval for the treatment.

Which training course?

Before embarking on any course, it may be useful to contact the AOC or the Institute of Complementary Medicine (see Chapter 1) for a list of accredited schools. Some schools offer courses that are aimed specifically at nurses. The Royal College of Nursing's Complementary Medicine Special-Interest Group may also have information about whether such courses are appropriate. There are also courses and seminars designed especially for nurses: details are available from the various aromatherapy organisations.

Recommended reading

- Davis, P. 1988. *Aromatherapy: an A–Z*. Saffron Walden: C. W. Daniel.
- Lawless, J. 1992. *The Encyclopedia of Essential Oils*. Shaftesbury: Element.
- Maury, M. 1990. *Marguerite Maury's Guide to Aromatherapy*. Saffron Walden: C. W. Daniel.
- Price, S 1991. *Aromatherapy for Common Ailments*. London: Gaia.
- Tisserand, R. 1990. *Aromatherapy for Everyone*. London: Arkana.
- Tisserand, R. 1992. *The Art of Aromatherapy*. Saffron Walden: C. W. Daniel.
- Valnet, J. 1992. *The Practice of Aromatherapy*. Saffron Walden: C. W. Daniel.
- Worwood, V. A. 1992. *The Fragrant Pharmacy*. London: Bantam.

References

- Buckle, J. 1992. Which Lavender oil? *Nursing Times* 88(32): 54–5.
- Davis, P. 1988. *Aromatherapy: an A–Z*. Saffron Walden: C. W. Daniel.
- Lawless, J. 1992. *The Encyclopedia of Essential Oils*. Shaftesbury: Element.
- MacKenzie, J. & M. Gallacher. 1989. A sweet-smelling success. *Nursing Times* 85(27): 48–9.
- NAHAT 1993. *Complementary Therapies in the NHS* (Research Paper No. 10). London: National Association of Health Authorities and Trusts.
- Tisserand, R. 1990. *Aromatherapy for Everyone*. London: Arkana.
- Wise, R. 1989. Flower power. *Nursing Times* 85(22): 45–7.

7 THERAPEUTIC TOUCH

Historical background

Healing by touch is a practice so ancient that it is impossible even to guess at when it was first practised; examples are found in cultures throughout the world, and it has never fallen into disuse.

People often think of this type of healing in spiritual terms – that a higher being's will is being channelled through the healer, and into the patient – but Therapeutic Touch (TT) seems to be closer to Eastern ideas of *prana*, a Sanskrit word which is difficult to translate, but which might be thought of as a regenerative energy found in all living creatures. The earliest writings on TT pay some attention to this idea, but later ones have tended to leave it out.

The roots of TT are found in studies carried out during the early 1960s into healing powers found in individuals, and the nursing model being developed by Martha Rogers in the USA. Bernard Grad, a Canadian biochemist, had met a healer called Oscar Estebany and invited him to spend a few weeks working under observation, in order that Dr Grad could extend his knowledge of the subject. Their partnership was to stretch out over several years. Grad compared the healing rates in artificial wounds in mice when Estebany treated them by touch, and when a person with no known healing powers did so. Estebany's mice healed faster (Grad *et al.* 1961).

At about the same time that Grad and others were undertaking their research, Martha Rogers, a professor in nursing at New York University, published her first work in what would she would develop into the 'Science of Unitary Man' (now 'Human Beings' – Rogers 1980). This is an extremely complex theory which has evolved over the years, but Jean Sayre-Adams, the leading exponent of Therapeutic Touch in the UK, has offered this concise three-part summary of the main points (1993):

- Human beings are energy fields – not *have* energy fields, but *are* energy fields.
- Humans and the environment are continually, simultaneously, and mutually exchanging energy with each other (environment refers to everything exterior to human, including other people).
- Universal order is a force innate to all energy fields.

Two elements were now in place; the third came when Dolores Krieger, an American nurse who had been intrigued by research into healing, met Dora Kunz, who is sometimes described as a 'sensitive'. Together they explored ways of harnessing the healing power they believed to be latent in everyone, and the technique they developed was christened 'Therapeutic Touch' by Dr Krieger. (The term 'Krieger-Kunz method' is sometimes used, but increasingly rarely.) About ten years later, Krieger found that her work dovetailed with that of Martha Rogers, providing a theoretical base that was firmly rooted in a nursing model.

Krieger published her first study, which appeared to demonstrate that TT raised haemoglobin levels in volunteers, in 1972, but it seems to have had no great impact, possibly because there were problems with the experimental design. She repeated the study under more stringent conditions two years later, and the paper she published in 1974 is now seen as seminal.

Therapeutic Touch has aroused a lot of interest in the USA, and is now taught in around eighty schools of nursing there; the National League for Nursing has also endorsed its use in practice. Acceptance in the UK has been slower, but the establishment of the Didsbury Trust in 1988 (see 'Resources'), where the technique can be learned by nurses, has led to a growth in interest.

The Trust set out, in 1993, to determine the approximate number of practitioners in this country, as no one can make more than a guess about how many there are.

Further reading

- Benor, D. J. 1990. Survey of spiritual healing research. *Complementary Medical Research* 4(3): 9–32.
- Courtenay, A. 1991. *Healing Now*. London: Dent.
- Krieger, D. 1979. *The Therapeutic Touch: how to use your hands to help or heal*. New York: Prentice Hall.

What is Therapeutic Touch?

Therapeutic Touch (TT) is a therapy which combines elements of Eastern philosophy, healing by 'laying on of hands', Martha Rogers' 'Science of Unitary Beings' (Rogers 1980), and concepts found in the branch of physics dealing with quantum mechanics.

The basic principle is that all living things are energy fields, which in turn are part of a greater field; individual fields interact, and a TT practitioner aims to use directed interaction to 'repattern' or 'rebalance' energy in the person whom they are treating, restoring the equilibrium which accompanies what we understand as 'health'.

TT has a unique position among complementary therapies, because it was chiefly developed by one nurse and has come to be closely associated with the nursing model developed by another.

Visiting a practitioner of Therapeutic Touch

As the experiments described on pages 92–3 illustrate, physical contact is not necessary for TT to be performed, although use of the word 'touch' suggests that it is essential. This has led to some difficulties in explanation of the theory.

With a few minor differences, most authors describe the following sequence, followed once the patient is in a comfortable position:

- **Centreing** The practitioner relaxes into a calm but alert state, sometimes using meditation or visualisation techniques to achieve this.
- **Assessment** The practitioner runs his or her hands above the patient's body, trying to sense subtle differences in the 'feel' of the energy field, but also using all his or her other senses to pick up other clues from the patient, on both a conscious and subconscious level.
- **Clearing** The hands are smoothly swept from head to toe, keeping just above the surface, to facilitate energy flow within the patient's field.
- **Intervention** In this phase, energy is actively rebalanced.
- **Evaluation** The practitioner relies on his or her judgement to know when the treatment is complete.

There is no set time that a treatment period is expected to last, nor is there a minimum or maximum number of treatment sessions.

When treatment is complete, the patient should feel rested and relaxed, while the practitioner may feel energised.

Further reading

– Macrae, J. 1992. *Therapeutic Touch: a practical guide*. New York: Alfred Knopf.

Indications

According to Jean Sayre-Adams there are *no* conditions in which TT might not play a part in alleviating or obviating symptoms.

Nurses working in the field of mental health have started looking at ways of introducing the technique into their work (Hill & Oliver 1993); Jean Sayre-Adams, who until recently believed that psychotic illnesses were a contra-indication to TT, now thinks that this may not be the case.

Dolores Krieger's 1979 book, *The Therapeutic Touch*, gives case histories covering conditions as varied as pain due to fractured ankle, rheumatoid arthritis, crying babies, and raised temperature. Research studies have looked at the value of Therapeutic Touch in anxiety, responses to stress in both newborn infants and adults, post-operative pain, and tension headaches; a paper published in 1993 invited discussion of the use of Therapeutic Touch in mental-health nursing (Hill & Oliver 1993).

Contra-indications

There are no apparent contra-indications to TT on physiological grounds, but a therapy that appears to some people as remarkably like spiritual or psychic healing, or 'laying on of hands', may offend deeply-held beliefs.

Caution must also be exercised if the patient has any mental-health problems, particularly psychotic illness; until further work is done in this area, the use of TT should be restricted to only the most experienced practitioners.

Research

Although Therapeutic Touch is, in comparison to the other therapies in this book, still in its infancy, a surprisingly large amount of methodologically sound research has been carried out. However, unlike most of the other therapies, it is not easy to obtain copies of original papers: many have been published in journals that are not widely available in the UK, such as *Subtle Energies* or *Psychoenergetic Systems*. Also, some of the larger studies currently exist only as doctoral theses in US university libraries, and are thus extremely difficult for British readers to get hold of.

Because it is so new a technique, it is important that anyone wanting to know more about it goes back to original sources, but they must be prepared for the possibility of a lengthy wait – and for a large bill for reprints! The Didsbury Trust published a collection of the more important original papers in 1994, and an updated textbook is in preparation.

If a full literature search is not feasible, there is a 1988 paper by Janet Quinn, in a reasonably easy-to-find journal, which critically reviews much of the research into the therapy in its first twelve years or so (Quinn, J. F. 1988. Building a body of knowledge: research on Therapeutic Touch, 1974–1986. *Journal of Holistic Nursing* 6(1): 37–45). As more research is undertaken in the UK, it should become easier to obtain published results.

Examples of research

The studies below give an idea of the sort of research that has been undertaken so far.

Alleviating tension headaches

A study of 60 volunteers with tension headaches divided the volunteers into two groups: half received TT, while the others received a placebo – the practitioner merely mimicked the movements of Therapeutic Touch, without 'centreing'. The subjects who received the treatment were more likely to have a reduction in pain, and this was greater and lasted for longer.

– Keller, E. & V. M. Bzdek 1986. Effects of Therapeutic Touch on tension headache pain. *Nursing Research* 35(2): 101–5.

Recovering from stressful experiences

A study involving 30 children, aged between two weeks and two years of age, found that Therapeutic Touch significantly reduced the time needed to calm them down after undergoing stressful experiences – such as having blood samples taken – compared with those who received 'casual' touch (patting and stroking).

– Kramer, N. A. 1990. Comparison of Therapeutic Touch and casual touch in stress reduction of hospitalized children. *Pediatric Nursing* 16(5): 483–5.

Wound healing

In this study, 44 young, healthy volunteers agreed to have incisions made on their arms; in addition to standard wound dressings, 23 received Therapeutic Touch, but, using an ingenious arrangement, the experimenters kept this secret from the subjects. On the sixteenth day, 13 of the TT group had healed wounds, while none of the controls did.

– Wirth, D. P. 1990. The effect of non-contact therapeutic touch on the healing rate of full-thickness dermal wounds. *Subtle Energies* 1(1): 1–20.

This experiment was replicated recently, and is described at length here as an all too rare example of the kind of well-designed research which can do so much to help the credibility of claims made for some therapies, by forestalling claims that results were due to suggestibility or placebo.

Full-thickness dermal wounds, using a 4 mm punch biopsy, were performed on the lateral deltoid muscles of 24 healthy volunteers, who were told that the experiment was about the use of a non-contact diagnostic device measuring 'biopotentials'. The physician performing the biopsies was also kept uninformed about the real purpose of the study. Wounds were treated with an antibacterial solution, then covered with an occlusive dressing.

Subjects were randomised into two groups, and asked to report, individually, to a laboratory each day. They were led by a person, also blinded to the experiment's purpose, to a chair by a one-way-mirror, behind which they believed was the diagnostic machine. For the treatment group, a TT practitioner was behind the mirror, and she performed TT for five minutes.

Dressings were changed on days 5 and 10, and on each occasion, they were assessed by the physician who inflicted the wounds. He looked at infection, re-epithelialisation, wound closure, scar formation, pigmentation, and cosmetic appearance. Photographs were also taken for assessment by three independent physicians, who were asked to rate the wounds as either 'fully healed' or 'not fully healed'.

On analysis, wound infection was left out of consideration due to 'insufficient data', and re-epithelialisation and wound closure were combined, as the clinical estimates were identical on days 5 and 10.

On day 5, five treated and twelve control subjects had unhealed wounds; on day 10, the figures were two and eight, respectively. The independent assessors showed high correlation with the experimental assessor's findings.

– Wirth, D. P., J. T. Richardson, W. S. Eidelman, *et al.* 1993. Full-thickness dermal wounds treated with non-contact Therapeutic Touch: a replication and extension. *Complementary Therapies in Medicine* 1(3): 127–32.

Implications for nursing

It has been suggested that 'the evidence shows that interest in and commitment to Therapeutic Touch has grown rapidly among clinicians for essentially one reason – it seems to work' (Sayre-Adams 1993). If the body of research evidence, showing significant advantages for both patients and practitioners, is to be believed – and most of it appears to be methodologically sound – then it appears that TT is worthy of further investigation.

However, sensitivity must be called for in the introduction of such a distinctly unorthodox treatment method. Firstly, TT appears, on the surface, almost indistinguishable from psychic, faith, or spiritual healing, in that one person is using some form of 'universal energy' in an attempt to induce physiological effects in another. The connection is spurious, as controlled trials in which the subject is unaware that TT is being used seemed to have ruled out the co-operative element essential to most forms of healing; but the patient may not always be in a position to think over such a fine point.

Secondly, because there simply is no way, as yet, of proving the existence of this postulated energy flow, it would be hard for a nurse to defend him- or herself, should a patient or client claim that harm had been done to them through the use of TT. There does seem to be a growing body of evidence that supports TT's claims, but it is still far from orthodox validation. 'Informed consent' is a tricky concept at the best of times, but when the theory behind a treatment is as far removed from 'accepted knowledge' as it is in TT, a whole range of problems presents itself.

Growing public and professional awareness of TT, and further research, will do a lot to resolve these difficulties; for the moment, though, nurses wishing to train in the technique should bear them in mind.

Resources

Training and regulation

There is no barrier to anyone reading something on TT, and then going on to practise it; relatively few nurses know a great deal about the technique at the moment, as it is so new, which makes it difficult to differentiate immediately between a skilled practitioner and an absolute beginner.

The Didsbury Trust (see below) set up the first of its accredited courses in Therapeutic Touch in 1992, in the hope of providing a standardised training; it is in the process of establishing a regulatory body for practitioners. The Trust is always interested in making contact with TT practitioners in the UK with whom it has not already established links, as there is no documented evidence for how widely used the therapy actually is.

The Trust, which was granted registered charity status in 1989, was set up to enhance nurses' 'natural skills and therapeutic abilities', as well as helping them to deal with the emotional needs created by the nature of nursing.

The Didsbury Trust
Sherborne Cottage, Litton, near Bath, Avon BA3 4PS.

Recommended reading

- Courtenay, A. 1991. *Healing Now*. London: Dent.
- Krieger, D. 1979. *The Therapeutic Touch: how to use your hands to help or heal*. New York: Prentice Hall.
- Macrae, J. 1992. *Therapeutic Touch: a practical guide*. New York: Alfred Knopf.

A new British text, bringing TT up to date, is in preparation. A source book of seminal papers is available from the Didsbury Trust.

References

- Grad, B., R. J. Cadaret & G. J. Paul 1961. An unorthodox method of treatment of wound healing in mice. *International Journal of Parapsychology* 2(1): 5–19.
- Hill, L. & N. Oliver 1993. Therapeutic Touch and theory-based mental health nursing. *Journal of Psychosocial Nursing* 31(2): 19–27.
- Krieger, D. 1972. The response of *in vivo* human hemoglobin to an active healing therapy by laying-on of hands. *Human Dimensions* 1(1): 12–15.
- Krieger, D. 1974. Healing by the laying-on of hands as a facilitator of bioenergetic change: the response of *in vivo* hemoglobin. *Psychoenergetic Systems* 1: 121–9.
- Krieger, D. 1979. *The Therapeutic Touch: how to use your hands to help or heal*. New York: Prentice Hall.
- Rogers, M. 1980. Nursing: a science of unitary man. In Riehl, J. & C. Roy (eds): *Conceptual Models for Nursing Practice*, 2nd edn. Norwalk, CT: Appleton-Century-Crofts.
- Sayre-Adams, J. 1993. Therapeutic Touch – principles and practice. *Complementary Therapies in Medicine* 1(2): 96–9.

8 NUTRITIONAL THERAPIES

Historical background

For as long as medicine has been practised, food has been recognised as providing more than nutritional needs. The original nutritional therapist was probably the first person who found that eating something made him or her feel better or worse, and passed the information on.

Over the centuries, different foodstuffs have been valued for their medicinal properties: according to one author, garlic was prescribed in ancient Egypt, Babylonia and Greece as a cure for many disorders, while cabbage was recommended by Hippocrates for cardiac problems, and was used as a wound dressing in 19th-century France (Olsen 1989). A more widely-known example is the administration of lime juice to British sailors in the 18th century, as prophylaxis for scurvy (scorbusis), which led to the slang term 'limey' (see Box 8.1). It was only in this century that the active ingredient in citrus fruits was isolated.

A Polish biochemist working in London, Casimir Funk, proposed in 1912 that there were substances in some foods, present in minute quantities, which were essential to life; he named them 'vital amines', or 'vitamines'. The first of these had actually been discovered twenty years earlier, and by 1915 several diseases had been found to be preventable if extracts from certain foods were given. Increasingly efficient analytic techniques made it possible to isolate the active substances, and the foundations were laid for the system we have today: the fat-soluble vitamins A, D, E and K, and the water-soluble B complex and C.

Many nutritional therapies were developed based on the use of these newly-identified substances, and later advances in scientific knowledge, like the discovery of possibly tissue-damaging 'free radicals', and the antioxidant properties of some vitamins, have led to claims that vitamin supplements may slow the ageing process (Passwater 1991).

Other nutritionally-based theories of health promotion in recent years have included the roles of minerals and micronutrients, dietary fibre, cholesterol and other lipids, food additives, 'complex' carbohydrates, and salt. A critical review of the evidence put forward for these theories, and several others, can be found in a book by Yetiv (1988).

Further reading

- Mayes, A. 1986. *The Dictionary of Nutritional Health – a guide to the relation between diet and health.* Wellingborough: Thorsons.
- Oliver, P & A. Peiser. *How Are You? – why 'normal' isn't normal.* London: Stenadelle.
- Truswell, A. S. 1992. *ABC of Nutrition,* 2nd edn. London: British Medical Journal.
- Walji, H. 1992. *Vitamin Guide: essential nutrients for healthy living.* Shaftesbury: Element.
- Yetiv, J. 1988. *Sense and Nonsense in Nutrition.* London: Penguin.

What are nutritional therapies?

Nutritional therapies is an umbrella term, covering a vast range of treatments and philosophies. For example, there are disciplines like nutritional medicine, defined as 'the study of the interactions of nutritional factors with human biochemistry, physiology and anatomy, and how the clinical application of a knowledge of these interactions can be used in the prevention and treatment of disease, as well as in the improvement of health' (Davies & Stewart 1987); and macrobiotics, 'the art of choosing food according to a set of principles, with the objective that man, in order to live naturally, actively and healthily, must eat natural foods' (Mayes 1986). The first of these does not seem too far removed from orthodox medicine; while the second, in which foods are classified according to their Yin and Yang characteristics, has elements which simply cannot be understood in terms of Western science.

These examples demonstrate how wide an area nutritional therapies covers, and it continues to expand, as the briefest examination of the shelves marked 'complementary medicine' in a large bookshop or library will show: authors with impressive credentials, and others with none, apparently promise to cure everything from coryza to cancer, by advising extra intake of some nutrients, or reduced intake of others, or both. If texts concerning slimming are included, it becomes almost impossible to keep up with the claims: diets that only burn up certain types of fat, or that will lead to weight loss in specific areas of the body leaving the rest unchanged, are just two that have challenged beliefs fundamental to 'orthodox' nutritional science.

Yet despite evidence that interest in nutritional therapies is growing, they received only a passing mention in the 1993 BMA report on complementary therapies; and the survey it contains – of which the authors say 'it is ... likely that the main therapies currently available in the UK are represented' – appears to have excluded them altogether. The reasons for this are not clear, but it may be a reflection of how nebulous the whole area has become.

Unlike all the other chapters in this book, then, this one will present only an overview of the subject. Readers wishing to find out more about specific therapies may find the 'Further reading' sections useful.

What follows is a small selection of only a few of the more widely-known nutritional therapies and diets. Any aimed solely at people wishing to lose weight have not been included because, however different they may appear, their underlying principle must always be the same: energy use should exceed energy intake.

Nutritional medicine

Davies and Stewart (1987) identify four factors that influence nutritional status:

- the quality of the food we eat;
- the quantity of the food we eat;
- the efficiency of digestion, absorption and utilisation;
- biochemical individuality.

Nutritional medicine aims to correct problems in one or more of these areas. So, for example, a therapist who believes that hyperactivity in a child might be due to chemical additives (such as colouring agents) or residues (such as pesticides) would be looking at food quality, when seeking a cause for hyperactivity. Yet each child is different, so biochemical individuality would also be a crucial consideration. An **exclusion diet** might be used here: the person fasts, or starts a fairly bland diet regime; if the symptoms subside, the likely cause is nutritional. Different foodstuffs can then be reintroduced, to identify those that trigger a reaction (Brostoff & Gamlin 1989).

Gerson therapy

The **Gerson therapy** (Holmes 1988), which its practitioners say has benefits for victims of cancer, arthritis, and many other conditions, is based on the theory that toxicity results from pollution, particularly in food, building up in the body; this affects the efficiency of digestion, causing alterations in the body's cells, these being related to biochemical individuality. The regime involves eating only organic vegetables, supplemented with hourly vegetable juice, or calves' liver juice; some dairy products may be added later. Coffee enemas, which practitioners believe will boost the liver's detoxification rate, are also given. The regime is an extremely time-consuming one, because of the time involved in finding the right kind of food, and preparing it.

Megavitamin therapy

Megavitamin therapy has been hotly debated for some years. Linus Pauling, a highly respected US chemist, became interested in vitamin C in the 1960s, and went on to develop a theory that an optimum mental state could be achieved biochemically, using substances like vitamins; to describe this state, he coined the adjective *orthomolecular*. Other researchers seized on this concept, and the disciplines of **orthomolecular psychiatry** and **orthomolecular medicine** were born.

Put simply, the idea behind megavitamin treatment is that, for some reason, the body cannot utilise enough of the vitamins in the diet, and deficiency results. To get round this, doses many times higher than the recommended daily minimum are given (Stanway 1992).

Pauling went on to claim that giving very high doses of vitamin C could prolong the life of terminally-ill cancer patients (Cameron & Pauling 1976), but the methodology used in the trial was claimed by others to have several problems which invalidated the results (Yetiv 1988).

Macrobiotics

Macrobiotics (from the Greek *macro*, large, and *bios*, life), starts from the principle that 'we first take an overview or holistic perspective about eating, and only then should we focus down on microscopic nutritional details' (Gulliver 1988). There are four main points:

- a person's diet should be based on staple foods, with supplementary and seasonal foods added;
- those foods should be whole and of local provenance, to provide balance between the person and his or her environment;
- different foodstuffs have different Yin and Yang qualities (see Chapters 4 and 13), which should be taken into account;
- the way those foods are cooked is of great importance (for example, microwave cooking is believed to have adverse effects on Qi within foods – Gulliver 1988).

Adults who follow macrobiotic diets will avoid many of the problems associated with the usual Western diet, but it has been suggested that children could suffer nutritional deficiencies (Mayes 1986).

Complementary nutritional therapy

Usually just called **nutritional therapy**, the adjective 'complementary' is sometimes added to avoid confusion with the blanket term used for all other treatments. The Society for the Promotion of Nutritional Therapy defines this as 'a therapeutic approach which aims to explore all possible avenues whereby a patient's nutrition can be manipulated to obtain maximum health promotion'.

When looking for the cause of a health problem, three possible diagnoses are examined:

- allergy or intolerance to food or environmental factors;
- toxicity arising from heavy metals or chemicals, because of environmental exposure, lowered eliminative ability, poor liver function, or any combination of these factors;
- deficits of nutrients because of insufficient intake, malabsorption, or 'special needs'.

One diagnosis does not, of course, exclude either or both of the others.

If any of these diagnoses can be made, provisionally, confirmation comes from a 'therapeutic trial', which involves education about nutrition, a modified diet, and, where necessary, nutritional supplements (Lazarides 1993).

Optimum nutrition

Optimum nutrition is based on three principles (Holford 1992):

- each person is biochemically unique, and therefore each person's nutritional needs are also unique;
- there is an intimate connection between nutrition and the environment;
- the human race's nutritional needs must be considered in the light of the fact that they have been shaped over many thousands of years.

Practitioners working on optimum nutrition lines believe that talking about 'recommended daily amounts' of vitamins and nutrients is not helpful, and say that four analyses – of diet, biochemical status, symptoms and lifestyle – can, when the results are collated, indicate whether an individual's diet is deficient in any way, and what supplements are necessary.

Indications

There are very few conditions which nutritional therapists feel will not benefit from their treatment. A brief list can be found in a book by Ward and others (1990), but much more detail is given by Davies and Stewart (1987), who use twenty-three broad headings under 'The nutritional management of some diseases and common ailments'; these include cardiovascular disease, problems with bones and joints, and disorders of the central nervous system.

Contra-indications

As every nurse knows, sound nutritional management is an essential part of care for every person. If the therapist is well-trained and qualified, there should be no contra-indications, because he or she will know when to give priority to 'orthodox' medical treatment.

A Swedish study (Bosstrom & Rossner 1990), looking at problems arising where 'alternative' therapies had supplanted conventional treatment, found that the majority of deaths or serious complications occurred when catabolic diseases had been treated by the institution of a vegetarian diet or regimes involving fasting.

Some nutritional supplements can interact with prescribed medication: for example, vitamin C (ascorbic acid) can increase the effects of salicylates (for example, aspirin), decrease the effects of some anticoagulants and psychoactive drugs, and exacerbate the side-effects of digitalis and some antibiotics. Even 'ordinary' foodstuffs can interfere with the pharmacokinetics of certain drugs (McPherson 1993). It is therefore extremely important that when a person seeking nutritional advice is having any concurrent medical treatment, his or her responsible medical practitioner should be kept informed of the therapy.

Research

A vast amount of research into different aspects of nutritional therapies has been carried out, particularly in recent years; critical analyses of the most important papers can be found in Yetiv's work (1988).

One research paper which led to a great deal of controversy in recent years concerned the Bristol Cancer Help Centre (BCCH; Bagenal *et al.* 1990). This establishment, set up in 1980, lays great emphasis on holistic care and counselling, and used to prescribe the 'Bristol Diet', a wholefood regime with vitamin supplements. A comparative study was set up, in which women at the BCCH were compared with others receiving treatment at three conventional centres. When the results were published in 1990, it seemed as though the BCCH was obtaining systematically *worse* results than the hospitals, but the interpretation of the results was challenged, and the dispute continues today (Buckman & Sabbagh 1993); see Chapter 17 for further discussion of this controversy.

BOX 8.1
A CONTROLLED TRIAL OF A NUTRITIONAL THERAPY

The first controlled trial of a nutritional therapy was probably that undertaken by James Lind in 1747. His account, reproduced in Truswell's book (1992), makes fascinating reading today:

On the 20th of May 1747, I took twelve patients in the scurvy, on board the *Salisbury* at sea. Their cases were as similar as I could have them. They all in general had putrid gums, the spots and lassitude, with weakness of their knees. They lay together in one place, being a proper apartment for sick in the fore-hold; and had one diet common to all ... Two of these were ordered each a quarter of cyder a-day. Two others took twenty-five guttae [drops] of *elixir vitriol* a-day, upon an empty stomach; using a gargle strongly acidulated with it for their mouths. Two others took two spoonsful of vinegar three times a-day, upon an empty stomach; having their gruels and their other food well acidulated with it, as also the gargle for their mouth. Two of the worst patients, with the tendons in the ham rigid ... were put under a course of sea-water. Of this they drank half a pint every day, and sometimes more or less as it operated, by way of gentle physic. Two others had each two oranges and one lemon given them every day. These they ate with greediness, at different times, upon an empty stomach. They continued but six days under this course, having consumed the quantity that could be spared. The two remaining patients, took the bigness of a nutmeg three times a-day, of an electuary recommended by an hospital-surgeon, made of garlic, mustard-seed, *rad. raphan.*, balsam of Peru, and gum myrrh; using for common drink, barley-water well acidulated with tamarinds ...

The consequence was, that the most sudden and visible effects were perceived from the use of the oranges and lemons; one of those who had taken them, being at the end of six days fit for duty ... The other was the best recovered of any in his condition; and being now deemed pretty well, was appointed nurse to the rest of the sick.

BOX 8.2
ALLERGIES

Food allergy is one of the most hotly debated issues in nutritional therapy today, yet until fairly recently, it was barely known outside specialist nutritional circles.

The explosion of consumer awareness has led to more and more people taking an interest in what they are eating; a similar upsurge in health awareness has resulted in growing demand for 'healthy' foods; and the extraordinary expansion of the environmental or 'green' movement has directly led to people wanting reassurance that their foodstuffs have not been contaminated with toxic substances, either deliberately – for example, with pesticides – or indirectly, through pollution.

The combination of these factors has caused a demand for information that is unprecedented in Western society, and the upshot has been that the possible existence of allergies to certain foodstuffs 'is at the interface between scientific immunology, food technology and quackery' (Davies & Stewart 1987).

At one extreme in this debate are those who believe that only organically-grown, pesticide-, preservative- and colouring-free, unprocessed foods should be eaten, while the opposite position is occupied by people – including many members of the medical profession – who dismiss it all as a passing fad. Members of this latter group have suggested that concern about food allergy is no more than another example of the 20th-century phenomenon of trying to avoid responsibility for problems, by laying the blame on extrinsic factors: '*your* child is a naughty brat, but *my* child's behaviour, on the other hand, is the result of hyperactivity triggered by an as yet unidentified dietary allergen'.

The debate has not been helped by loose usage of terminology by all sides in discussion, but in 1984, the Royal College of Physicians and the British Nutrition Foundation produced a report which has helped clarify what, exactly, constitutes 'food sensitivity', and this has been developed by other authors. Truswell (1992) suggests the following definitions:

- **Food sensitivity** is a reproducible, unpleasant reaction to an identifiable part of the diet, which affects one person but not another. This can be divided in two:
  - **(Chemical) food intolerance** is where the response can be evoked under double-blind conditions (see Chapter 17);
  - **Food aversion** includes psychological and psychosomatic reactions.

- Each of these further subdivides:
  - *Food intolerance* includes **food allergy**, where there is an immunological reaction, and '**other types of food intolerance**', where a foodstuff may be an irritant, have a pharmacological action on the individual, cause problems because of the lack of a normally present enzyme in the body, or simply cause problems for no known reason.
  - *Food aversion* includes **psychological food intolerance**, where the reaction does not occur if a person is given the supposed trigger unknowingly, and **food avoidance**, where the sole cause is psychological.

Despite the plethora of books on the subject, and the work which has been done in centres like Great Ormond Street, London, and Addenbrookes Hospital, Cambridge, no reliable figures appear to exist at present for the incidence or prevalence of chemical food intolerance. It is to be hoped that a balanced picture will eventually emerge, but at present, the claims and counterclaims being made have rendered objective discussion very difficult.

Further reading

- Brostoff, J. & L. Gamlin 1990. *The Complete Guide to Food Allergy and Intolerance*. London: Bloomsbury.
- Davies, S. & A. Stewart 1987. *Nutritional Medicine*. London: Pan.

Implications for nursing

Sue Holmes, a senior lecturer in nutrition, has said: 'Nutrition must be seen as an integral part of total care. It should be regarded as a positive contribution to treatment. Its success or failure is largely dependent on the nurse's interest, knowledge and understanding' (Holmes 1993). Because many nutritional therapies may interfere with 'orthodox' treatment, such knowledge is vital.

If a patient or client has been receiving some form of nutritional therapy before he or she comes into a nurse's care, it is important that this be discussed with medical staff, pharmacy staff and a dietitian, as the person may wish to continue the regime alongside other prescribed treatment.

With the explosion of interest in 'healthy eating' in recent years, members of the public have a wealth of information sources on which they can draw; but unfortunately not all of these are without ulterior motives for the messages they promote. Nurses are trusted to give unbiased information, which means that they have a duty to be as well informed as possible about a subject which affects every patient or client they will ever have in their care; as interest in nutritional therapies grows, they need to ensure that their own information sources are trustworthy.

As one author has pointed out, when trying to obtain information about everyday foodstuffs, 'it is important to know who the financial sponsors of any organisation are. If they are supported by companies who make money out of less nutritious foods their advise needs to be taken with caution. This applies to the British Nutrition Foundation which advises the government about nutritional policy, yet is itself funded by the major companies producing confectionery, high-fat foods, processed meats, food chemicals and alcohol' (Holford 1992). Sadly, similar caution may have to be exercised in dealing with organisations and individuals promoting certain supplements; as another author warns (Foulkes 1991), anyone considering a career in the area of nutrition should, when checking out a training establishment, find out whether or not 'you really are [to be] trained as an independent professional practitioner and not as a salesman for supplements. If the training organisation actually recommends its own range of vitamins, minerals, and so on, what is the relationship between the course and the products?'

During the preparation of this chapter, several people from different areas of practice commented on the problem of getting unbiased advice, but none was prepared to give any comments on the record. For the moment, then, all that can be said is that nurses wishing to know more about the subject need to look very critically at the claims made by any organisation; for although the vast majority of practitioners undoubtedly have only their patients' or clients' interest at heart, it is the tiny minority who could do most to discredit the practice of real therapists.

Resources

Training and regulation

The Institute for Complementary Medicine (see Chapter 1) has a division devoted to nutritional therapies, and will provide all the necessary information individuals may want about a particular therapy, the qualifications of practitioners, and establishments offering training.

Recommended reading

- Bray, G. A. & D. H. Ryan (eds) 1993. *Vitamins and Cancer Prevention* (Pennington Centre Nutrition Series, No. 3). Baton Rouge/London: Louisiana State University Press.
- Brostoff, J. & L. Gamlin 1990. *The Complete Guide to Food Allergy and Intolerance*. London: Bloomsbury.
- Davies, S. & A. Stewart 1987. *Nutritional Medicine*. London: Pan.
- Holmes, P. 1988. The Gerson therapy. *Nursing Times* **84**(14): 41–2.
- Mayes, A. 1986. *The Dictionary of Nutritional Health*. Wellingborough: Thorsons.
- Oliver, K. & A. Peiser 1991. *How Are You? – why 'normal' isn't normal*. London: Stenadelle.
- Passwater, R. A. 1991. *The New Supernutrition*. New York: Pocket Books.

- Pauling, L. 1986. *How to Live Longer and Feel Better*. New York: W. A. Freeman.
- Ward, B., P. Tripp & M. Evans 1990. *Your Diet*. Bromley: Harrap.
- Yetiv, S. 1988. *Sense and Nonsense in Nutrition*. Harmondsworth: Penguin.

References

- Bagenal, F. S., D. F. Easton, E. Harris, *et al.* 1990. Survival of patients with breast cancer attending Bristol Cancer Help Centre. *Lancet* **2**: 606–10.
- Bostrom, H. & S. Rossner 1990. Quality of alternative medicine – complications and avoidable deaths. *Quality Assurance in Health Care* **2**(2): 111–17.
- British Medical Association 1993. *Complementary Medicine: new approaches to good practice*. Oxford: Oxford University Press.
- Brostoff, J. & L. Gamlin 1990. *The Complete Guide to Food Allergy and Intolerance*. London: Bloomsbury.
- Buckman, R. & K. Sabbagh 1993. *Magic of Medicine? An investigation into healing*. London: Macmillan.
- Cameron, E. & L. Pauling 1976. Supplemental ascorbate in the supportive treatment of cancer: prolongation of survival times in terminal human cancer. *Proceedings of the National Academy of Science* **73**: 3685.
- Davies, S. & A. Stewart 1987. *Nutritional Medicine*. London: Pan.
- Foulkes, J. 1991. *Complementary Medicine Careers Handbook*. Sevenoaks: Headway.
- Gulliver, N. 1988. Macrobiotic diet. In Rankin-Box, D. (ed.): *Complementary Health Therapies: a guide for nurses and the caring professions*. London: Chapman & Hall.
- Holford, P. 1992. *Optimum Nutrition*. London: ION Press.
- Holmes, P. 1988. The Gerson therapy. *Nursing Times* **84**(14): 41–2.
- Holmes, S. 1993. Building blocks. *Nursing Times* **89**(21): 28–31.
- Lazarides, L. 1993. Personal communication, June.
- Mayes, A. 1986. *The Dictionary of Nutritional Health*. Wellingborough: Thorsons.
- McPherson, G. 1993. Absorbing effects. *Nursing Times* **89**(32): 30–2.
- Olsen, K. 1989. *The Encyclopedia of Alternative Health Care*. London: Piatkus.
- Passwater, R. A. 1991. *The New Supernutrition*. New York: Pocket Books.
- Royal College of Physicians/British Nutrition Foundation 1984. Food intolerance and food aversion. *Journal of the Royal College of Physicians* **18**(1): 2.
- Stanway, A. 1992. *Alternative Medicine: a guide to natural therapies*. London: Bloomsbury.
- Truswell, A. S. 1992. *ABC of Nutrition*, 2nd edn. London: British Medical Journal.
- Ward, B., P. Tripp & M. Evans 1990. *Your Diet*. Bromley: Harrap.
- Yetiv, J. 1988. *Sense and Nonsense in Nutrition*. London: Penguin.

9 HYPNOTHERAPY

Historical background

Hypnosis as a *medically* useful technique seems to be, in comparison to some of the other therapies discussed in this book, a relatively modern one, dating back only to the late 18th century. However, there is evidence that rhythmic dancing and drumming, which can induce states indistinguishable from those now associated with hypnosis, have a long history in Africa and North America, while several authors mention the use of hypnotic techniques in ancient Egypt, in ancient Greece, and, in Britain, by the Druids, although they do not give specific references for these assertions (Lesser 1989).

The first recorded accounts of something very close to what would now be recognised easily as hypnotism were performed in the latter half of the 18th century by a Germany physician, Franz Anton Mesmer (1734–1815). He believed that there was an invisible fluid or force permeating the universe that could also be found in the human body: 'a fluid universally diffused, so continuous as not to admit of a vacuum, incomparably subtle, and naturally susceptible of receiving, propagating, and communicating all motor disturbances' (cited in Winn 1958). This force could be acted upon within the human body, where it became subject to the force of two magnetic poles, Mesmer believed, and he called this manifestation 'animal magnetism'.

In his first case, he gave an iron preparation to a female patient with uncontrollable, 'hysterical' symptoms, and sought to redirect the flow of 'animal magnetism' by the application of magnets to her body. The treatment was successful, and soon became popular; he sought further fame by moving his practice from Vienna to pre-revolutionary Paris, where there was a large number of wealthy women who suffered from '*les vapeurs*'.

Mesmer's fame grew so much, and 'mesmerism' became so popular, that he was forced to devised group treatments: patients sat around a large tub, filled with a mixture of water, powdered glass and iron filings, holdings metal rods which passed through the lid of the tub, to rest in the fluid. Mesmer then 'magnetised' the contents of the tub, and played soothing music while the patients – up to fifteen at a time – passed through a kind of crisis, ranging from shaking to convulsions, from which they emerged feeling better (Trotter 1975).

A Royal Commission was set up, under the chairmanship of Benjamin Franklin, by Louis XVI to examine mesmerism, and its findings, published in 1774 – that although Mesmer had undoubtedly effected some cures, 'animal magnetism' could not be demonstrated – led to Mesmer's being denounced as a charlatan. He was to die penniless.

But mesmerism did not die with him. Some physicians seemed to think that there was something worth investigating in the demonstrable effects of the technique, and there were occasional reports of trance states being used for anaesthetic purposes.

In 1843, a Scots surgeon working in Manchester, James Braid, published a book called *Neurhypnology*, which sought to reclaim mesmerism for use in medicine, by providing an explanation of the phenomenon which would satisfy the scientifically inclined. Braid repudiated the idea of animal magnetism, for a start, but argued that the trance state was genuine enough, and declared that it could be induced in a variety of ways: for example, by getting the subject to stare at a bright object. What was happening, he said, was simply a neurological response to a stimulus; and to distance his theory even further from mesmerism, he coined the word 'neurhypnotism' (from the Greek *hypnos*, meaning sleep) to describe it (Inglis 1979). This would later be shortened to 'hypnotism'.

Braid's ideas were taken up by W. B. Carpenter, who held the chair in physiology at London University; he believed that many phenomena exhibited by hypnotised subjects could be explained in terms of sensory hyperacuity and muscular hyperactivity. In the meantime, James Esdaile, a Scots surgeon employed by the East India Company in Calcutta, employed a mesmerist to put patients into a trance before he operated on them, with considerable success, and J. B. Dods developed Carpenter's work in the United States.

Hostility remained, however: the British Association for the Advancement of Science refused a paper on hypnosis from Braid, and a professor of medicine named Elliotson resigned his chair at University College Hospital, London, because of a total ban on mesmerism there (Zangwill 1987b).

Another setback, according to Inglis (1979) was the first demonstration of ether's anaesthetic properties in the US, in 1846: '… and when Robert Lister performed the first operation with an anaesthetic in Britain his comment, "this Yankee dodge beats mesmerism hollow", reflected the relief which surgeons felt that they would not, after all, have to learn a technique which they had resisted so long, and so vehemently'.

After Braid's death in 1860, interest in hypnotism dwindled, but it was rekindled during the 1880s when Braid's work appeared in French and German for the first time, and the greatly respected French neurologist, Jean-Martin Charcot, declared that hypnotism had a valuable part to play in the treatment of hysteria. A great deal of work was done in Europe, concentrating on examining the effects of hypnosis on bodily functions not normally under conscious control, while medical practitioners in Britain tended to stay aloof, even after a British Medical Association inquiry in 1891 found that the phenomena described in much of the literature were genuine (Zangwill 1987a).

While European studies continued – most famously, in the early work of Sigmund Freud, who was to give up its practice but who retained a lifelong interest – the subject seemed to languish in Britain and the United States, until a psychologist at Yale, C. L. Hull, started undertaking rigorous research into the subject during the 1930s.

Since then, hypnotherapy has fought a long uphill battle towards scientific respectability, which it appears to be winning, Hypnotism is a recognised therapeutic tool, but its unfortunate associations with quackery and entertainment have left it largely outside the mainstream of medicine, despite the recommendations of bodies such as the Britain and American Medical Associations that it be included in all pre-registration courses.

Further reading

- Hartland, J. 1971. *Medical and Dental Hypnosis*. London: Baillière Tindall.
- Inglis, N. 1979. *Natural Medicine*. London: Collins.
- Lesser, D. 1989. *The Book of Hypnosis*. Birmingham: Curative Hypnotherapy Examination Committee.
- Olsen, K. G. 1991. *The Encylopaedia of Alternative Health Care: a complete guide to choices in healing*. London: Piatkus.
- Stanway, A. 1992. *Alternative Medicine: a guide to natural therapies*. London: Bloomsbury.
- Winn, R. B. 1958. *Scientific Hypnotism*, 2nd edn. London: Thorsons.

What is hypnotherapy?

Hypnotherapy is, by definition, a treatment which involves the use of hypnosis: but that begs the question, what is hypnosis? Hypnosis is the induction of a trance-like state, in which the person becomes more compliant, relaxed, and open to suggestion, and in which long forgotten memories may be brought back to consciousness.

(Contrary to popular belief, though, not everyone will 'regress', as some memories are simply too painful to be exhumed, and this technique requires a great deal of trust on the client's part.) It is possible to implant suggestions that can be triggered after the person has come up of the trance, but – again contrary to popular belief – it is probably impossible to make someone do anything against his or her wishes, even if it were ethically permissible to do so. Physiological changes may be seen and measured in the hypnotised person: for example, parts of the body can be anaesthetised, and levels of hormones produced under stress can be lowered appreciably.

Hypnotherapy, then, is the use of hypnotic techniques in the treatment of some conditions with a large psychological component. It is an accepted part of many medical practitioners' and dentists' therapeutic repertoire, but it has yet to successfully shake off the aura of mystery, tinged with suggestions of charlatanism, that has for so long surrounded it in the public eye.

As with many phenomena associated with the brain, no one can say for certain how hypnosis works, but there is no doubt that it is a natural part of the mind's function. Probably everyone has experienced trance-like states at certain times in their life, most commonly when bored; motorway driving, in which a person discovers they have safely travelled for several miles but cannot remember anything about it, is an oft-quoted example. Another one with which many people will be familiar is the experience in the classroom in childhood, when the teacher rudely awoke them from a reverie with a question, and there was a moment of panic as they realised they did not know what had been happening for a few minutes before – and then mysteriously, the correct answer to the question appeared from some recess of the mind, proving that at least some part of it *had* been paying attention.

It has been suggested that there is a distinct area in consciousness, lying somewhere on the line between being fully awake and completely unconscious, which is entered when the person is hypnotised; the fact that electroencephalograms (EEGs) show a unique pattern in the hypnotised subject is seen as supporting this theory.

Visiting a hypnotherapist

The first appointment is a trust-building exercise; unless a rapport develops between client and therapist, the all-important 'therapeutic relationship', which is vital to successful treatment, will not be established.

In some cases, it may be necessary to spend time on dispelling myths about what hypnotherapy actually is, and what it can do; many clients have odd preconceptions about the treatment.

The therapist will collect as much information about the person as possible, looking at all aspects of his or her life, and possible roots of the problem which led the person to seek help. No moral judgements are made, as these are not the practitioner's concern.

Induction, the process of relaxing into the hypnotic state, is started by the client getting comfortable on a chair or couch, possibly covered with a light blanket, as the body temperature may fall during hypnosis; the therapist then talks the client through a series of exercises that aid relaxation. Very few practitioners use dangling watches or flashing lights, as the voice alone should be sufficient, but the client's expectations may need to be fulfilled, if treatment is going to be successful. This applies particularly to children, and many therapists will keep a watch or something similar in a desk drawer, for use if necessary.

Caution must be exercised in the choice of images used in relaxation. One therapist recalled asking a girl to imagine herself under a tree, beside a smoothly flowing river, with a field of corn waving gently in the breeze. The visualization was so successful that it triggered an attack of hay fever.

Once the hypnotic state has been reached, the client is often encouraged to look at the problem, and to seek insight into it by recalling long buried thoughts and memories from the past. The unconscious mind is thus recruited into the effort to overcome the problem. As mentioned above, there may be insuperable resistance to such **regression**, but the therapist can use formulae to ensure that the block does not extend too far for meaningful material to be unearthed: for example, 'you will recall as much as it is safe for you to recall at this time'.

Not all conditions need this approach, though; **suggestion therapy**, where there may be no need to seek the cause, is of use in giving up smoking, calming exam nerves, wart removal, and several other problems.

Many clients will be taught how to induce the state themselves, to help with relaxation. The therapist may provide tapes to help with this.

The number of sessions required depends on the person, the nature of the problem, and the way he or she responds to the therapy.

Further reading

- Tamin, J. 1988 Hypnosis. In Rankin-Box, D. (ed.): *Complementary Health Therapies: a guide for nurses and the caring professions*. London: Chapman Hall.

Indications

One of the areas in which hypnotherapy has recorded many successes is in the treatment of physical conditions where they may be a large psychological element, particularly stress: migraines, skin problems like eczema and psoriasis, and some problems with the gastro-intestinal tract, such as colitis, irritable bowel syndrome, and constipation, are just a few examples.

Insomnia and anxiety frequently respond to skilled hypnotherapy, and people suffering with phobias, obsessions, some addictions and dependency states, undesirable habits and compulsions (for example, smoking and compulsive gambling) can benefit from the therapy.

A specialised area of therapy is the treatment of sexual problems, such as impotence. Vaginismus may respond to hypnotherapy.

Relaxation is an important part of hypnotherapy, and patients undergoing potentially distressing procedures can be helped to endure them more comfortably (see the 'Research' section).

These are just a few examples of where hypnotherapy can be of use; more complete lists can be found in the books listed under 'Recommended reading'.

Contra-indications

When a health problem is purely physical, such as an acute infection, hypnotherapy has no direct part to play in treatment, although in some cases it may help with the alleviation of symptoms. A person with severe psychological health problems, such as someone in deep depression or in a psychotic state, might possibly be further disturbed by attempts to induce a hypnotic state. With this exception, when a skilled hypnotherapist is consulted, there are no contra-indications to treatment; if the therapist cannot help, he or she will say so, and will suggest where appropriate treatment might be found. Should there be any doubt at all, a medical check-up will be recommended, and most hypnotherapists are advised, during training, always to consider this as a matter of course.

As one writer put it, 'hypnosis is like a gun – it's not the tool itself, but the operator who makes it dangerous' (Olsen 1991).

Research

There is a vast body of research into hypnotherapy, and two journals exist, published in the UK, which are devoted to the subject: the *British Journal of Experimental and Clinical Hypnosis*, now called

Contemporary Hypnosis, which has been established for some years, and a more recent one, the *European Journal of Clinical Hypnosis.* Trials of interest to nurses and midwives include the following.

With chemotherapy

In a comparison of children aged between 10 and 19 receiving chemotherapy, it was found that those taught self-hypnosis and relaxation vomited less (two-thirds did not vomit at all) than the children who did not receive instruction in the technique; they were also able to maintain a higher fluid intake.

– Cotanch, P., M. Hockenberry & S. Herman 1985. Self-hypnosis as antiemetic therapy in children receiving chemotherapy. *Oncology Nursing Forum* 12(4); 41–6.

As analgesia in labour

In a randomised trial, women who were taught self-hypnosis for analgesia in labour did not apparently have less need for painkillers than women in the control group, but they were much more likely to be satisfied with their delivery. An unexplained side-effect seemed to be that their pregnancies were prolonged by a few days.

– Freeman, R. M., A. J. Macaulay, L. Eve, *et al.* 1986. Randomised trial of self-hypnosis for analgesia in labour. *British Medical Journal* 292: 657–8.

With hyperventilation

Two studies were carried out in the cardiac department of Charing Cross Hospital in London, following the observation that patients who hyperventilated could be helped back to a normal breathing pattern by using hypnosis. Some of these patients, though, would 'flip' back into hyperventilation for no apparent reason.

The researchers found that of the 60 patients studied in two trials, a third would hyperventilate when stressful episodes in their lives were recalled under hypnosis, although physiological screening for the likelihood of this happening had apparently cleared them. They suggested that hypnosis could be used to identify 'at risk' patients and their individual stressors, enabling care and medical interventions to be planned with a higher degree of safety.

– Conway, A. 1989. Hypnosis and research into mind/body relationships. *Complementary Medical Research* 3(2): 9–11.

In A&E departments

Examples of how hypnotic techniques were used to help patients attending accident and emergency departments, particularly those who were in neurological shock, and how the need for analgesia was lessened, are given by two US nurses in a paper published in the nursing press.

– Puskar, K. & K. Mumford, 1990. The healing power. *Nursing Times* 86(33): 50–2.

Implications for nursing

Any technique that produces relaxation will be of value to patients, and nurses whose work involves counselling – especially some community psychiatric nurses – have used hypnosis successfully for some time.

There are many potential applications within other areas, for example in surgical units, where hypnosis might be a useful alternative to premedication, and could help in pain relief, and in units where uncomfortable procedures like sigmoidoscopies are performed.

Perhaps the most useful application of all would be if nurses could learn self-hypnosis as a counter to the high stress levels that are unavoidable in the profession.

However, to a lot of people, the idea of being hypnotised is unwelcome (although 'relaxation', which is in some ways indistinguishable from facets of hypnotherapy, is perceived as non-threatening). Beliefs still persist about the therapist being able to get their clients to do anything they want them to, although no evidence exists for this, and at some stages hypnotists have perpetuated myths about swivel-eyed Svengalis inveigling the unwary into performing exhibitionistic acts against their will.

The occasional story in the press or on television about 'hypnotherapists' who have assaulted their clients does little to reassure the public about their safety; few of those reports point out that anyone can put an advertisement in the paper, offering hypnotherapy, and that impressive-looking – but essentially valueless – certificates and 'diplomas' can be obtained, or even run up at the printer's shop, without any form of legal check; or that anyone can set up a 'training school', offering postal courses and entitling 'graduates' to put a string of letters after their names (see 'Training and regulation'). Public exposure may have little effect, though; when the BBC *Watchdog* programme took a very critical look at a 'therapist' whose practices were questionable, advertisements for his courses still appeared in a national newspaper on the following Sunday. As a result, a well-tested therapy, which could help with the resolution of existing problems, and the prevention of potential ones, is being under-used.

Nurses are in a position to help do something about this state of affairs. By becoming better informed about the subject, and liaising with colleagues and other health-care professionals who are using hypnosis in their work, members of the profession can allay the fears of patients and clients who want to know more about how hypnotherapy could help them. Perhaps there are enlightened managers who might utilise part of their training budgets to get nurses onto appropriate courses; only good could come from training staff members in a technique which could not only help them to help patients and clients, but which has the potential to help nurses help themselves. In the meantime, too many people may be being denied a therapy with a proven record in helping resolve stress-related disorders – and nurses, more than anyone, know how widespread such problems are.

Resources

Training and regulation

Anyone can call him- or herself a hypnotherapist, and reports of malpractice appear with sad frequency in the media. Establishing a therapist's credentials is not always easy; in 1990, one journal reported that 'there are 87 different organisations, not all reputable or discriminating, whose initials could be used after the practitioner's name' (Marsh, A. 1990. Hypnotherapy. *Which? Way to Health* (October), 160–1). That figure is now nearer a hundred.

The Institute of Complementary Medicine (see Chapter 1) maintains a register of hypnotherapists who belong to professional organisations which the ICM recognises, and this register is available to the public. Perhaps more importantly, the ICM can also advise on the value of qualifications claimed by practitioners.

There are many reputable organisations, one of which was named in the 1993 BMA report:

National Council of Psychotherapists
46 Oxhey Road, Oxhey, Watford WD1 4QQ.

There is a bewildering range of courses available, from those offering tuition by post through to intensive courses; these last are more likely to qualify successfully students for inclusion on a reputable register. Before registering as a student on any course, it is advisable to seek advice first from a professional organisation.

Recommended reading

- Hartland, J. 1971. *Medical and Dental Hypnosis*. London: Baillière Tindall.
- Lever, R. 1988. *Hypnotherapy for Everyone*. Harmondsworth: Penguin.
- Markham, U. 1987. *Hypnosis*. London: Macdonald Optima.
- Young, P. 1987. *Personal Change Through Self-Hypnosis*. London: Angus & Robertson.

References

- British Medical Association 1993. *Complementary Medicine: new approaches to good practice*. Oxford: Oxford University Press.
- Inglis, B. 1979. *Natural Medicine*. London: Collins.
- Lesser, D. 1989. *The Book of Hypnosis*. Birmingham: Curative Hypnotherapy Examination Committee.
- Marsh, A. 1990. Hypnotherapy. *Which? Way to Health* (October), 160–1.
- Olsen, K. G. 1991. *The Encyclopaedia of Alternative Health Care: a complete guide to choices in healing*. London: Piatkus.
- Stanway, A. 1992. *Alternative Medicine: a guide to natural therapies*. London: Bloomsbury.
- Trotter, W. R. 1975. *Man the Healer*. Hove: Priory Press.
- Winn, R. B. 1958. *Scientific Hypnotism*, 2nd edn. London: Thorsons.
- Zangwill, O. L. 1987a. Hypnotism, history of. In Gregory, R. L. (ed.): *The Oxford Companion to the Mind*. Oxford: Oxford University Press.
- Zangwill, O. L. 1987b. Mesmerism. In Gregory, R. L. (ed.): *The Oxford Companion to the Mind*. Oxford: Oxford University Press.

10 HOMOEOPATHY

Historical background

The term 'homoeopathy' is derived from the Greek words *homoios* (like) and *patheia* (suffering). In fact, it was Hippocrates was who first developed the idea that an agent that can cause a disease might also be used to treat it. Paracelsus, too, in the early 16th century, made references to such a concept.

Certainly the idea of treating like with like is not new. Many folk remedies were selected using this principle: rubbing the feet with snow to relieve chilblains, for example, or using stinging nettles to treat the pain and swelling of rheumatism.

But it was the work of a German doctor, Samuel Hahnemann (1775–1843), that established homoeopathy as a coherent system of medicine. Hahnemann had become increasingly concerned about the medicine of his day and its appalling effects on patients. Bleeding by leeches, cupping and venesection were still common, as were violent purges and the use of toxic substances such as mercury in 'treatments' for many diseases.

So concerned was he that he gave up his practice, and worked instead as a translator of medical texts. While translating a materia medica by William Cullen, a Scottish physician, Hahnemann became intrigued by Cullen's explanation for the effectiveness of quinine as a treatment for malaria. Cullen posited that its success lay in its astringent properties. Hahnemann was unconvinced by this and went on to inject himself with quinine. He began to experience the symptoms of malaria – a result which was the exact opposite to the ways remedies were thought to work. The symptoms disappeared as soon as Hahnemann stopped taking the quinine.

In an essay entitled 'A New Principle for Ascertaining the Curative Powers of Drugs and some examinations of the Previous Principles', written in 1796, Hahnemann gave his own explanation – that the substance which cured someone of a disease actually produced the same symptoms in a healthy individual *'similia similibus* – likes with likes'.

Hahnemann went on to test other drugs on healthy volunteers, 'provers' as he called them, cataloguing the effects. Many of the drugs were poisons, so when Hahnemann tested them on patients he tried diluting them as much as possible. It was then that he found that the more dilute the drug, the stronger its curative effects became. By 1810 Hahnemann had published a materia medica of the medicines he had 'proved' and an explanation of his theories in one of his most famous works, *The Organon of Medicine* (1810).

In 1813 he had the opportunity to treat homoeopathically 180 soldiers suffering from typhoid after the battle of Leipzig. Only one patient died, and Hahnemann gained much respect as result. Hahnemann continued to research homoeopathic remedies and to offer them to patients until his death in 1843.

Homoeopathy was first practised in Germany and France, but it spread to Britain and the United States in the 19th century. In 1844 the American Institute of Homoeopathy was founded. The American Medical Association (AMA) was founded three years later – specifically to oppose the homoeopaths, whom physicians and the American pharmaceutical companies saw as a threat to conventional medicine. They waged a vicious campaign against homoeopaths until the end of the century, including forbidding AMA members to prescribe homoeopathic remedies or to have anything to do with homoeopaths. Ironically, homoeopathy continued to flourish in America until, in 1930, the AMA suddenly did an about-face and invited homoeopaths to join them, an invitation they accepted. From this point on, the practice of homoeopathy in the USA began to decline.

The doctor who introduced homoeopathy to Britain in the 19th century was Frederick Hervey Foster Quin, who also became physician to Prince Leopold of Saxe-Coburg, uncle of Queen Victoria. In fact, homoeopathy has now received the patronage of the royal family for six generations.

In 1844 Quin went on, despite opposition from orthodox practitioners, to set up the British Homoeopathic Society, which is now known as the Faculty of Homoeopathy.

In the 19th century homoeopathy hospitals were built, and during the 1854 outbreak of cholera, mortality figures for the Royal London Homoeopathic Hospital were 16.4 per cent, compared with an average of 51.8 per cent for all other London hospitals.

During the late 19th century and early 20th century two homoeopaths, Wilhelm Schuessler and Edward Bach, developed new types of treatment based on homoeopathic principles: mineral tissue salts and Bach flower remedies (see pages 135 and 138 respectively).

When the NHS was created in 1948 the homoeopathic hospitals entered the new health service, although this led to their offering orthodox as well as homoeopathic treatments. Homoeopathy is still available on the NHS, and in recent years there has been an upsurge in interest among medical practitioners. There are over six hundred doctors in the register of the Faculty of Homoeopathy, and more than two thousand GPs are using some homoeopathy or referring patients to homoeopathic centres.

Further reading

- Campbell, A. 1984. *The Two Faces of Homoeopathy*. London: Jill Norman & Hobhouse.
- Cook, T. M. 1987. *Samuel Hahnemann: the Founder of Homoeopathic Medicine*. Wellingborough: Thorsons.
- Nicholl, P. 1988. *Homoeopathy and the Medical Profession*. London: Croom Helm.

What is homoeopathy?

Homoeopathy is a system of medicine based on the principle that 'like cures like'. In this system, a substance that *causes* symptoms in a healthy person can *cure* the same symptoms when they occur as part of a natural disease in a sick person. A good example is the treatment of eczema. It is well known that petrol and oil can cause cracks and itchiness in sensitive skin exposed to them. These symptoms are similar to those found in people suffering from eczema, and one of the homoeopathic remedies used to treat irritant eczema uses petroleum.

Hahnemann also found that the more *dilute* the drug, the *stronger* the effect, and therefore recommended that remedies should be administered in the smallest possible doses – an application of the idea of the 'minimum dose'. He experimented with more and more dilute solutions to the point at which the level of dilution was such that no molecules of the original substance could be found. Hahnemann claimed nevertheless that these extraordinarily dilute remedies had profound effects, provided that they went through an additional process of vigorous shaking or **succussion** at each stage of dilution. This process came to be known as **potentization**.

During his researches Hahnemann noticed that some of his patients had recurrent patterns of disease which did not respond to the indicated remedies. Hahnemann's explanation of these inherited systemic weaknesses and susceptibilities to particular illnesses was his theory of **miasms**. He identified three, and considered them to be the underlying cause of chronic diseases. These miasms were:

- **psoric miasm**, 'the itch' – Hahnemann believed this was an almost universal miasm;
- **syphilitic miasm**, passed from one generation to another;
- **sycotic miasm**, an inherited miasm due to gonorrhoea.

Today homoeopaths have identified other miasms, which are due to the effects of pollution, vaccines, drugs, and other diseases such as tuberculosis and cancer. In such cases, homoeopaths often use deeper-acting remedies, including some made from disease tissue of the corresponding miasm – for examples from gonorrhoeal pus 'medorrhinum', or from cancer tissue 'carcinocin'. These remedies are called **nosodes**.

Hahnemann also looked at what maintained a healthy body. He concluded that there is a **vital force**. When this force is confronted with a stimulus or stress stronger than itself, symptoms of illness are manifested in the body as the body tries to heal itself. Homoeopaths seek to redress this imbalance in the vital force to allow the body to heal itself completely.

There are more than two thousand homoeopathic remedies in use, and new remedies are still being developed. They are made from a very wide range of things: plants, animal products, insects, reptiles, minerals, metals, and chemical compounds.

First the substance has to be prepared so that potentization can be undertaken. The way this is achieved depends on the nature of the substance. Methods include:

- *Preparing a tincture* A plant or part of a plant is gathered at the optimum time (usually spring or summer) and washed. The juice is extracted and added to absolute alcohol. (The proportion of juice to alcohol varies according to the plant.) The resulting solution is called the **mother tincture**.
- *Trituration* If the substance to be prepared is insoluble, it is ground for three hours with a specified amount of milk sugar (lactose), using a sterile pestle and mortar. This reduces the substance to the millionth dilution (6c or 30c potency), at which point the substance is soluble in water.

Most remedies that you can buy over the counter come in either 6c or 30c potency, but there are many other levels of potency which a trained homoeopath can use. The 'c' after the number refers to the way the remedy was diluted: the **centesimal scale** of dilution. In this, 1 drop of the tincture is added to 99 drops of distilled water or alcohol and vigorously shaken; this gives the first potency. This process is repeated by taking 1 drop of the previous potency and adding it to 99 drops of dilutant until the desired potency is achieved.

Some remedies may have a 'd' or an '×' after the number, which refers to the **decimal scale**. In this method the same process is used except that 1 drop of substance is added to 9 drops of alcohol or distilled water.

Homoeopathic remedies come in a variety of forms: tinctures, pilutes, tables, triturations, granules or powders. The remedy can be placed under the tongue, put into water and sipped, or put on a lactose tablet and then dissolved in the mouth.

As Hahnemann's original 'provings' were carried out using single substances, homoeopathic remedies are usually given as single remedies in single doses. A homoeopath then observes the patient's response and decides whether to wait, repeat the dose, choose a stronger dose, or change the remedy completely.

With acute conditions, one normally notices a change after the first dose. Chronic conditions, however, take longer to treat. A remedy should not be taken once an improvement has been noted. If the condition being treated is acute, remedies can be taken at half-hourly intervals, the intervals being increased as improvement occurs. Remedies should be taken at least 10–15 minutes after eating, and no food or strong-tasting drink ingested immediately after taking a remedy.

Remedies should be stored away from direct sunlight, in a cool, dry cupboard. They also should not be stored near strong-smelling substances. Remedies last for many years – some researchers suggest fifty or more.

Further reading

- Richardson, S. 1988. *A Guide to Homoeopathy*. London: Hamlyn.
- Vithoulkas, G. 1983. *Homoeopathy, Medicine for the New Man*. New York: Arco.
- Weiner, M. & K. Goss 1982. *The Complete Book of Homoeopathy*. New York: Bantam.

Visiting a homoeopath

The first appointment is likely to last about an hour. In order to treat anything successfully with homoeopathy, a practitioner must prescribe the right remedy and the right dosage for each patient. To do this, the homoeopath will ask many questions about the patient's illness, the health of his or her family (past and present), personal likes or dislikes, and the patient's physical and emotional temperament.

The homoeopath will want to hear about anything that might help establish the right remedy. As the Society of Homoeopaths (see 'Resources') encourages, 'Do not be afraid to mention something that you think is unusual or unimportant, and please help by giving accurate information'. All information is treated in strict confidence.

Patients should also tell their homoeopath about any medication they are already taking and about any planned dental treatment. Although homoeopathic remedies do not interfere with conventional medication, strong drugs like steroids, antibiotics and narcotics can mask symptoms. This can make the selection of a remedy more difficult, or can be an antidote to the remedy.

Once a patient has been given a homoeopathic remedy to take, he or she should also check back with the homoeopath before taking any new medication, in case this interferes with the action of the homoeopathic remedy, and vice versa.

The homoeopathic remedy prescribed will usually be in the form of pills which are put under the tongue and allowed to dissolve. It is important not to put anything else in the mouth for 10–15 minutes before or after taking the remedy, including things like toothpaste or cigarettes. Patients are also likely to be advised not to drink coffee or to take any sort of peppermint, eucalyptus oil, camphor or menthol, as these appear to undermine the effect of homoeopathic remedies.

Once a patient has taken a homoeopathic remedy he or she may experience a period of well-being and optimism, although some people actually find their symptoms get *worse* for a short time. If this happens, it is a normal part of the recovery process. Patients should make a note of any other symptoms experienced, as the homoeopath will want to discuss these at the next appointment. How quickly a homoeopathic treatment works depends on what is being treated; some can be very rapid in their effects, others more long-term. But as the Society of Homoeopaths points out, 'Be patient; it is much better for you to be cured of both the cause of your illness and its symptoms, rather than merely to relieve the symptoms.'

Like other complementary therapists, homoeopaths will also discuss other lifestyle issues that may be affecting a patient's health, and may suggest dietary or other lifestyle changes.

Indications

Homoeopathy as a system of medicine has been used to treat adults, children, animals and plants. It is also used as a complement to orthodox medicine, for example in helping the body cope with the effects of surgery.

Hahnemann grouped diseases into two categories, chronic and acute, both of which groups are claimed to respond well to homoeopathy. Homoeopathy also claims success where orthodox treatment has failed, for example with the common cold. Allergies, hayfever, asthma and eczema too can be treated homoeopathically.

In pregnancy and childbirth there is a wide range of homoeopathic remedies for problems such as morning sickness, breathlessness, swollen ankles and heartburn, as well as for speeding up labour and healing the perineum. Such remedies have the advantages of being both safe and without side-effects. Postnatally, homoeopathic remedies have been used to help with breastfeeding problems, depression, and incontinence.

The gentle nature of homoeopathy makes it a popular choice in the treatment of babies and children. Colic, teething problems, minor infections and colds can all be treated homoeopathically.

More serious conditions, such as cancer and arthritis, have also been treated homoeopathically; and at the London Lighthouse, an AIDS hospice, homoeopathy is being used to treat people with AIDS. At the other end of the spectrum, homoeopathy has also been used to help with nervous conditions such as exam nerves or fear of flying.

Homoeopathic remedies are used to prevent infection in cases of epidemics such whooping cough or typhoid. This is usually achieved using nosodes prepared from the bacteria or virus causing the infection.

There are no toxic side-effects from the use of homoeopathy, so most homoeopaths agree that homoeopathic remedies can, in many cases, be used by untrained individuals (see Box 10.1). Many homoeopathic pharmacies sell homoeopathic first-aid kits. However, it is important that professional help is sought if any symptom persists.

Self-help and homoeopathy

Although there are homoeopathic remedies that can be used safely by untrained individuals, they should not be offered to patients unless the member of staff has appropriate training, and permission from the patient and the patient's doctor has been given.

According to Otto Wolff (1991), for example, one of the most effective homoeopathic treatments in the early stages of colds, influenza and other feverish illnesses is Aconitum napellus 4× (most shops will only sell 6× or 30×, which will work just as well), 5 drops at hourly intervals, or, even better, in the compound preparation Infludo, taken as directed, hourly to begin with. Gelsemium 4× or 6× helps to relieve headaches and aching limbs. He also suggest adding Melissa comp. to hot lemon drinks to help the body heal itself.

Homoeopathic remedies are often recommended as treatment in first aid for shock and physical trauma (see Box 10.1).

BOX 10.1
HOMOEOPATHY AND FIRST AID

Homoeopathic remedies are ofen recommended as first-aid treatment for shock and physical trauma. Homoeopath Jonathan Stallick (1990) offers the following suggestions:

Arnica Injuries of all kinds, including post-operative trauma, should heal more quickly and less painfully if this is administered. Arnica also eases the general shock to the system. Use the 6th or 30th potencies in the form of tablets repeated hourly to six-hourly depending on severity. The ointment is good for bruised but unbroken skin. Midwives will find the 30th potency repeated three times daily for a few days helps bruising after childbirth.

Calendula Known as the homoeopathic antiseptic. Use as ointment, cream or tincture (dilute approximately 1 to 20) on broken skin and wounds to speed healing and relieve pain. Can be obtained in combination with Hypericum which adds to its pain-relieving properties. Use the tincture, diluted, as a mouthwash after dental operations.

Hypericum For use where parts full of nerves are affected, such as fingers and toes – for instance, fingers trapped in a door or any injury or trauma where there are severe shooting nerve pains. Use the 30th potency. Also useful for painful post-operative stitches.

Staphysagria Helps to relieve cystitis after operations, also painful post-operative stitch pains when Hypericum and Arnica fail.

Urtica urens Use for minor burns and bee stings. Can be taken in tablet form (6th or 30th potency) or applied in the form of a proprietary homoeopathic burn cream. For more severe burns, Cantharis, in tablet form, is worth trying (and, in any case, Arnica is worth giving to counteract the shock).

Carbo veg Often useful for wind in the upper abdomen occurring after abdominal operations.

Other useful homoeopathic self-help remedies include the following:

- *For tiredness* Two or three doses of Arnica 30c for sleeplessness after excessive physical effort; and Phosphoric acid (6×) up to three times a day for a week should help restore lost energy after long periods of strain or study.
- *For stress* Nux vomica 40 is useful for those who are overworking.

Further reading

There are a large number of homoeopathic self-help books on the market. Examples include:

- Castro, M. 1990. *The Complete Homoeopathy Handbook: a guide to everyday health care*. London: Macmillan.
- Cummings, S. & D. Ullmann 1986. *Everbody's Guide to Homoeopathic Medicines*. London: Victor Gollancz.
- Harland, M. & G. Finn 1991. *The Barefoot Homoeopath*. Clanfield, Hampshire: Hyden House.
- MacEoin, B. 1992. *Homoeopathy*. Dunton Green, Kent: Headway Lifeguides (Hodder & Stoughton).
- Shepherd, D. 1982. *Homoeopathy for the First-aider*. Saffron Walden: Health Science Press.

Contra-indications

Homoeopathic remedies are extremely safe, but situations in which their use would be unlikely to be helpful are those where permanent tissue damage has occurred, where there is a mechanical obstacle to recovery, such as a displaced vertebra, or where the patient has received a great deal of orthodox medicine to the extent that it is difficult to distinguish the original symptoms from the side-effects produced by the drug therapy. Even in such situations, however, homoeopathy can safely be used as a complement to orthodox treatment.

Research

There is now a body of evidence to support the existence of a homoeopathic effect. For example, two particularly significant trials were undertaken at the NHS Glasgow Homoeopathic Hospital.

One was a double-blind trial of homoeopathy in treating rheumatoid arthritis. Patients receiving homoeopathy remedies experienced a significant improvement, whereas those receiving a placebo experienced no significant change.

- Gibson, R. G., S. L. M. Gibson, A. D. MacNeill, *et al.* 1980. Homoeopathy therapy in rheumatoid arthritis: evaluation by double-blind clinical therapeutic trials. *British Journal of Clinical Pharmacology* 9(5)· 413–19

In the second, patients receiving homoeopathic treatment for hayfever showed a significant reduction in symptoms scores (as recorded by both the patient and the doctor) as compared with those receiving a placebo. It is noted in the research report that 'No evidence emerged to support the idea that placebo action fully explains the clinical response to homoeopathic drugs'.

- Taylor-Reilly, D., C. McSharry, M. A. Taylor, *et al.* 1986. Is homoeopathy a placebo response? *The Lancet* 2(8512): 881–5.

Another interesting study was published in 1984 by a veterinarian, Christopher Day, who found that Caulophyllum reduces stillbirths in pigs (a common occurrence in sows) by 10 per cent.

- Day, C. E. I. 1984. Control of stillbirths in pigs using homoeopathy. *Veterinary Record* 114: 216.

In Germany, a major research project is under way investigating the efficacy of a variety of complementary medicines, including homoeopathic remedies. The German Research Ministry (BMFT) has invested 10 million Marks (about £4 million). The findings will help health insurance companies decide which treatments they should pay for.

Useful articles for those interested in finding out more about homoeopathic research include these:

- Knipschild, P. 1991. Clinical trials of homoeopathy. *British Medical Journal* 302: 316–21.
- Righetti, M. 1992. Information on research in homoeopathy – where to get it. *Homoeopathic Links* 1: 35–6.

Not everyone accepts such evidence. In 1991, for example, Kleijnen *et al.* reviewed the quality of 107 controlled trials of homoeopathy in 96 published reports. They concluded that the evidence of clinical trials is positive but not sufficient to draw definite conclusions: most trials were, in their view, of low methodological quality.

- Kleijnen, J., P. Knipchild & G. ter Riet 1991. Clinical trials of homoeopathy. *British Medical Journal* 302: 316–23.

A more positive review of homoeopathic research is to be found in the following paper:

- Taylor-Reilly, D. & M. A. Taylor 1988. The difficulty with homoeopathy: a brief review of principles, methods and research. *Complementary Medical Research* 3(1): 70–8.

There are also surveys of the use of homoeopathic remedies. In one study, 73 doctors who practise homoeopathy were surveyed. Of these, 49 worked in general practice, 34 in private practice, and 15 in out-patient clinics. A total of 7218 consultations were given during the week of the survey, 88 per cent as part of the NHS. Some 35 per cent overall, and 25 per cent of general-practice consultations, were managed using homoeopathic medicine. These were combined with conventional drugs in 8.5 per cent of the prescriptions.

– Swayne, J. M. D. 1989. Survey of the use of homoeopathic medicine in the UK health system. *Journal of the Royal College of General Practitioners* (December) **39**: 503 6.

Other research reports on homoeopathy include the following:

– Brigo, B. 1991. Homoeopathic treatment for migraines: randomised double-blind controlled study of 60 cases. *Berlin Journal of Research in Homoeopathy* **1**(2): 98–106.
– Carey, H. 1986. Double-blind clinical trial of Borax and Candida in the treatment of vaginal discharge. *Committee of the British Homoeopathy Research Group* **15**: 12–14.
– Davey, R. W. 1990. Screening tests to antibacterial substances in plant extracts. *Complementary Medical Research* **4**: 1–5.
– Gibson, G. R., S. L. M. Gibson, A. D. MacNeill, *et al.* 1980. Homoeopathic therapy in rheumatoid arthritis: evaluation by double-blind clinical therapeutic trial. *British Journal of Clinical Pharmacology* **9**: 453–9.
– O'Neill, V. A. 1988. Challenger or charlatan? An overview of homoeopathy. *Complementary Medical Research* **3**(1): 70–8.
– Pinsent, R. J. F. H., G. P. I. Baker, G. Ives, *et al.* 1986. Does Arnica reduce pain and bleeding after dental extraction? *Committee of the British Homoeopathy Research Group* **15**: 3–11.
– Reilly, D. T. 1992. Hay fever and asthma trials. *Homoeopathy Today* **12**(8): 12–14.
– Shipley, M., H. Berry, G. Broster, *et al.* 1983. Controlled trial of homoeopathic treatment of arthritis. *Lancet* **1**: 482.

The problem is that very few of the two thousand or so homoeopathic remedies have been investigated. A homoeopath will generally not be able therefore to prove that a particular homoeopathic remedy taken for a particular problem by a particular individual will be effective. All we can say is that research has shown a homoeopathic effect, and if a homoeopath is properly qualified he or she is able to establish which homoeopathic remedy is likely to be effective in any given situation.

Implications for nursing

A MORI survey (1989) found that 80 per cent of patients using homoeopathy were satisfied with the results, and 75 per cent of those asked thought that alternative medicine should be available on the NHS.

In fact homoeopathy is available on the NHS. There are also five NHS homoeopathic hospitals in the UK (see 'Resources'). Nurses should be aware that in addition to the homoeopathic hospitals in the NHS, the family health service authorities have lists of homoeopathic doctors, broken down into regional and district health authorities. The British Homoeopathic Association (see 'Resources') can also supply lists of homoeopathic GPs (on receipt of an SAE).

A patient must live within the catchment area of the NHS homoeopathic GP in order to be included on the doctor's NHS list. However, most homoeopathic GPs will offer consultations on a private basis to patients living outside the area. There is no set scale of fees for a private consultation, but doctors can sign forms for private insurance companies.

Nurses also work in the NHS homoeopathic hospitals. As senior nurse Hilary Jenkins at the Royal London Homoeopathic Hospital (and a member of the council of the British Homoeopathic Association) has said, 'nursing homoeopathic patients is fundamentally no different from nursing patients being treated in other ways' (Dopson 1988).

There are also nurses who have become homoeopaths. For example, health visitor and homoeopath Kate Diamantopoulo runs a children's clinic in Brighton, where her patients are treated homoeopathically. She believes she can treat, with homoeopathy alone, 90 per cent of the children who are brought to her. The remaining 10 per cent she treats homoeopathically in conjunction with conventional medical treatment. Parents bring children to the clinic for help with some of the painful or chronic conditions that the medical profession can do little about except hand out yet more antibiotics or another cream: colic, asthma, eczema, and infections of the ear, nose or throat (Wade 1991).

The Natural Medicines Society (see Chapter 1) launched a campaign in 1992 to encourage the use of homoeopathic medicines by GPs. The Society argues that 'Homoeopathic medicine is the only complementary medicine "built into" the NHS: any doctor can prescribe it'. They claim that 'each year, over 750,000 homoeopathic prescriptions are written by doctors. The average homoeopathic prescription item costs at least 20p less than conventional prescriptions, and prescriptions also require 12% fewer items. If those GPs who now use no homoeopathic medicines followed the lead of GPs who do, the saving on the NHS drug bill would be at least £70 million a year'. A wider discussion of this argument is to be found in an article by Swayne (1992). Certainly a growing number of doctors are interested in training in homoeopathy – as far back as 1988 the Faculty of Homoeopathy reported a 50 per cent increase in the doctors they were training.

Four years of lobbying by Lucinda Ward, a retired nurse and member of the British Homoeopathic Association (BHA), resulted in the opening of a homoeopathic clinic at the Victoria Cottage Hospital in Sidmouth, Devon, in April 1992 – funded by the BHA. When it opened, senior nurse Malcolm Beebee said, 'This is a service the population wants.' In its first six months of operation, the clinic attracted out-patient referrals from 22 of the local GPs and had appointments booked six months in advance. The clinic had been scheduled to be held once a month, but this was soon increased to three times a month.

An analysis of the first six months (personal communication) showed that 52 per cent of patients attending were aged 60 years and over, and that 76 per cent were female. Interestingly, 38 per cent had had the illness or complaint that had precipitated the visit for more than ten years, and 68 per cent for more than two years. The most common reasons for attendance were musculo-skeletal conditions including osteoarthritis and rheumatism (24 per cent) and digestive disorders such as irritable bowel syndrome (17 per cent). Other conditions included mental-health problems such as anxiety and depression, allergies, skin complaints, neurological disorders, and circulatory problems. Scrutiny of individual cases demonstrated improvements and patient satisfaction was high.

When the term of BHA funding comes to an end it is hoped that the health authority will take over.

Another co-operative venture with which the BHA has been involved is the publication of *Homoeopathy for Midwives (& Pregnant Women)* which was written by Peter Webb (1992), in consultation with midwives from The John Radcliffe Infirmary, Oxford. Following publication, a research project involving pregnant women and the use of homoeopathic medicine was initiated. Certainly some midwives, especially independent midwives, are familiar with the use of homoeopathic remedies in pregnancy, and have incorporated them into their practice (Swinnerton 1990a & b, 1991a & b).

In 1993 the National Association of Health Authorities and Trusts published the findings of a national survey (NAHAT 1993) of district health authorities (DHAs), family health services authorities (FHSAs) and GP fundholders (GPFHs): this examined purchasers' attitudes towards the availability of complementary therapies in the NHS. More than 70 per cent of FHSAs and GPFHs, and 65 per cent of DHAs, were in favour of some or all complementary therapies being available on the NHS – free at the point of contact. Of those purchasers who felt that some complementary therapies should be available on the NHS, 60 per cent of DHAs thought homoeopathy should be available, as did 50 per cent of GPFHs and 65 per cent of FHSAs. Seven health-promotion clinics offering homoeopathy have been approved by FHSAs.

Most homoeopaths would agree that there are conditions requiring first aid which nurses could treat with only a basic knowledge of the principles of homoeopathy, but that chronic disease requires the skills of a trained homoeopath. However, nurses should gain permission from their employers before using any homoeopathic remedies.

Since July 1993, every Boots the Chemist has employed a 'consultant' to advise customers on homoeopathic remedies for common ailments. The Faculty of Homoeopathy (see 'Resources') helped draw up a training package for the thousand or so counter staff who have been become 'consultants'.

Certainly the sale of homoeopathic remedies is unlikely to be restricted either by the government or the European Union. The EU's homoeopathic directive, agreed in 1992, is a mandatory piece of EU legislation which requires member states to set up a system for the registration and approval of homoeopathic products on the market in accordance with guidelines it lays down, or to accept the decisions of other member states on homoeopathic products, thus allowing their importation and sale without restriction.

Resources

National Health Service homoeopathic hospitals

Bristol Homoeopathic Hospital
Cotham Road, Cotham, Bristol BS6 6JU.

Glasgow Homoeopathic Hospital
1000 Great Western Road, Glasgow G12 0RN.

Department of Homoeopathic Medicine
Mossley Hill Hospital, Park Avenue, Liverpool L18 8BU.

The Royal London Homoeopathic Hospital
Great Ormond Street, London WC1N 3HR.

Tunbridge Wells Homeopathic Hospital
Church Road, Tunbridge Wells, Kent TN1 1JU.

Homoeopathic suppliers

Many chemists and health food shops stock a limited range of homoeopathic remedies. The following are specialist pharmacies or manufacturers. Orders can be supplied by post.

Ainsworths Homoeopathic Pharmacy
38 New Cavendish Street, London W1M 7LH.

Buxton & Grant
176 Whiteladies Road, Bristol BS8 2XU.

Freeman's
7 Eaglesham Road, Clarkston, Glasgow G76 7BU.

Galen Homoeopathics
Lewell Mill, West Stafford, Dorchester, Dorset DT2 8AN.

Goulds
14 Crowndale Road, London NW1 1TT.

Helios Homoeopathic Pharmacy
97 Camden Road, Tunbridge Wells, Kent TN1 2QR.

P. A. Janssen
The Pharmacy, 28 Ampthill Road, Bedford MK42 9HG.

Jolleys Pharmacy
36 Witton Street, Northwich, Cheshire CW9 5AH.

Nelson's Homoeopathic Pharmacy
73 Duke Street, Grosvenor Square, London W1M 6BY.

Weleda (UK) Ltd
Heanor Road, Ilkeston, Derbyshire DE7 8DR.

Other items

Other homoeopathic supplies, such as phials, unmedicated tablets and storage boxes, are available by post from:

The Homoeopathic Supply Company
4 Nelson Road, Sherringham, Norfolk NR26 8BU.

Training and regulation

Registers of both medical doctors who have become homoeopaths (from the Faculty of Homoeopathy) and homoeopaths without a medical background (from the Society of Homoeopaths) are available.

Society of Homoeopaths (SH)
2 Artizan Road, Northampton NN1 4HU.

The Society is a registering body for professional homoeopaths in the UK. Registration is possible after graduating from an accredited college, plus a minimum of one year's clinical supervision, a review of a patient case, and a one-day site visit to observe the applicant in practice. Members must abide by the Society's code of ethics and practice. The Society has a list of practitioners, which is available on receipt of a large SAE. The Society also runs various postgraduate training courses and seminars, promotes research into homoeopathy, and has various information leaflets, and audio tapes.

British Homoeopathic Association (BHA)
27a Devonshire Street, London W1N 1RJ.

The BHA was founded in 1902 and is linked to the Faculty of Homoeopathy; membership is open to anyone interested in homoeopathy. It has the largest lending library of homoeopathic books in the country open to the general public (subject to membership). The Association also has a mail-order book service, produces information leaflets on homoeopathy, has an information service, produces a bi-monthly journal, and puts on lectures and seminars throughout the country.

The BHA is keen to make links with the nursing profession and to set up courses for those interested in becoming homoeopaths. The BHA can supply lists of homoeopathic doctors and pharmacies, on receipt of a large SAE.

The Faculty of Homoeopathy, The Royal London Homoeopathic Hospital
Great Ormond Street, London WC1N 3HR.

Other useful addresses

British Institute of Homoeopathy (BIH)
Victor House, Norris Road, Staines, Middlesex TW18 4DS.

Hahnemann Society (HS)
Humane Education Centre, Avenue Lodge, Bounds Green Road, London N22 4EU.

Homoeopathic Development Foundation (HDF)
10 Church Street, Steeple Bumpstead CB9 7DG.

Homoeopathic Trust for Research and Education (HTRE)
2 Powis Place, London WC1N 3IIT.

International Podiatric Association of Homoeopathic Medicine (IPAHM)
134 Montrose Avenue, Edgware, Middlesex HA8 0DR.

Register and Council of Homoeopathy (RCH)
243 The Broadway, Southall, Middlesex UB1 1NF.

UK Homoeopathic Medical Association
243 The Broadway, Southall, Middlesex UB1 1NF.

Colleges

The major homoeopathic training colleges are banding together to form the Organisation of Independent Homoeopathic Colleges, which will be seeking accreditation.

The following list of training colleges is not comprehensive, but may help in selecting an appropriate course. Before embarking on any course, nurses should take advice from their professional associations.

College of Homoeopathy (CH)
Regents College, Inner Circle, Regents Park, London NW1 4NS.

College of Practical Homoeopathy (CPH)
422 Hackney Road, London E2 7SY.

Hahnemann College of Homoeopathy (HCH)
243 The Broadway, Southall, Middlesex UB1 1NF.

London College (LC)
7a Gilmore Road, London SE13 5EY.

London College of Classical Homoeopathy (LCCH)
c/o Morley College, 61 Westminster Bridge Road, London SE1 7HT.

London School of Classical Homoeopathy (LSCH)
57 Wise Lane, Mill Lane, London NW7 2RN.

For enquiries and concerning further education, write to:

The Vice-Principal,
London School of Classical Homoeopathy, Otteley, Oddington, Kidlington, Oxford OX5 2RA.

Northern College of Homoeopathic Medicine (NCHM)
First Floor, Swinburne House, Swinburne Street, Gateshead, Tyne and Wear NE8 1AX.

Scottish College of Homoeopathy (SCH)
17 Queens Crescent, Glasgow G4 9BL.

Recommended reading

– Blackie, M. 1984. *The Challenge of Homoeopathy: the patient not the cure*. London: Unwin.
– Hahnemann, S. 1810 *The Organon of Medicine*, reprinted 1983. London: Victor Gollancz.
– Harland, M. & G. Finn 1991. *The Barefoot Homoeopath*. Clanfield, Hampshire: Hyden House.
– Lessell, C. 1983. *Homoeopathy for Physicians*. Wellingborough: Thorsons.
– Lockie, A. 1989. *The Family Guide to Homoeopathy*. London: Elm Tree Books.
– Pratt, N. 1991. *Homoeopathic Prescribing*. Beaconsfield, Buckingham-shire: Beaconsfield Publishers.
– Richardson, S. 1988. *A Guide to Homoeopathy*. London: Hamlyn.
– Shepherd, D. 1989. *Homoeopathy for the First Aider*. Saffron Walden: C. W. Daniel.
– Smith, T. 1982. *Homoeopathic Medicine: a doctor's guide to remedies for common ailments*. Wellingborough: Thorsons.
– Speight, P. 1990. *Homoeopathy for Emergencies*. Saffron Walden: C. W. Daniel.
– Speight, P. 1992. *Homoeopathy: a home prescriber*. Saffron Walden: C. W. Daniel.
– Ullmann, D. 1991. *Discovering Homoeopathy*. Richmond, California: North Atlantic Books.
– Ullmann, D. 1988. *Homoeopathy: medicine for the 21st century*. Richmond, California: North Atlantic Books.
– Vithoulkas, G. 1981. *The Science of Homoeopathy*. New York: Grove Press.
– Vithoulkas, G. 1983. *Homoeopathy: medicine for the new man*. New York: Arco.
– Vithoulkas, G. 1985. *Homoeopathy*. Wellingborough: Thorsons.
– Weiner, M. 1989. *The Complete Book of Homoeopathy*. New York: Avery.
– Wright, Hubbard, E. 1990. *Homoeopathy as Art and Science*. Beaconsfield, Buckinghamshire: Beaconsfield Publishers.

Mineral tissue salts

In 1873 a German homoeopathic physician called Wilhelm Schuessler published the results of his research into the effects of certain **mineral salts** on the body. He believed that many diseases and conditions resulted from imbalances of these minerals in the body: if cell balance were restored, a cure would be effected. Schuessler identified twelve vital mineral salts which he believed could be used singly or in combination to treat these cell imbalances.

The salts are prepared in homoeopathic doses, whereby the active ingredient is diluted with lactose. With mineral salt remedies the proportions are 9 parts lactose to 1 part active mineral salt. The mixture is ground together and a further dilution is undertaken with 9 parts lactose to 1 part of the mixture. With each dilution, the potency of the remedy is increased. Most remedies are sold at 6× potency.

According to Peter Gilbert (1989), a doctor and expert on mineral salt therapy, 'Mineral tissue salt therapy is directed at an illness. Diagnose the illness by recording the symptoms and then administer the mineral tissue salt or combination of mineral tissue salts that has been found to correct the cellular imbalances causing the symptoms to occur. It is therefore very well suited to the self-treatment of common family ailments.'

The twelve single tissue salts, and the ailments they can be used in treating, are given below:

- **No. 1 Calc. Fluor.** (calcium fluoride) Deficient tooth enamel; flabbiness (including hernias and prolapse); late development of teeth in infants and children; over-relaxed tissues; piles; poor teeth; varicose ulcers; varicose veins.
- **No. 2 Calc. Phos.** (calcium phosphate) Bony deformities; chilblains; children outgrowing their strength; chronic tonsillitis; coccydynia; coldness; cramps; delay in teething, and general teething problems; hypochondriasis (with No. 6 Kali. Phos.); liability to colds and catarrh; polypus; poor nutrition and digestion; slow healing of fractures; some skin diseases (catarrhal type); some types of anaemia.
- **No. 3 Calc. Sulph.** (calcium sulphate) Boils; catarrh; dandruff; falling hair; frontal headaches (especially among older people); gum boils; kidney upsets; liver upsets (with No. 11 Nat. Sulph.); neuralgia; pancreatic upsets; pimples (during adolescence); skin eruptions; skin slow to heal; sore lips; vertigo with nausea.
- **No. 4 Ferr. Phos.** (iron phosphate) All minor respiratory disorders; chestiness (in alternation with No. 5 Kali. Mur. 6×); childhood illnesses; chills (feverishness); congestions; coughs and

colds; excessive periods; first stages of inflammations and fevers; haemorrhage; inflammatory rheumatism; nosebleed; throbbing congested headaches.

- **No. 5 Kali. Mur.** (potassium chloride) Acne; burns; catarrh; chestiness (in alternation with No. 4 Ferr. Phos. 6× for children's feverish colds); chickenpox; cold symptoms; constipation (in pregnancy or in liverish states); coughs; diarrhoea (from eating fatty foods); eliminating side-effects of immunisation or vaccination if given in advance; eczema (particularly infantile); leucorrhoea; menorrhagia (but check with a doctor first); minor respiratory disorders; measles; mumps; piles; scalds; scarlet fever; second stage of inflammation of all '-itis' illnesses; shingles; warts; wheeziness; white/grey coating of tongue.
- **No. 6 Kali. Phos.** (potassium phosphate) Alopecia; despair; emotional strain; excessive blushing; fearfulness; being highly strung; hysteria, loss of mental and nerve power; incontinence or retention of urine from nervous causes; ineffectual labour pains; anxiety; melancholia; menstrual colic (spasms, cramps, etc.); nervous asthma; nervous debility; nervous diarrhoea; nervous headache; nervous indigestion; neuritis; nightmares and phobias; sexual incompetence and frigidity; temporary nerviness; timidity; shyness.
- **No. 7 Kali. Sulph.** (potassium sulphate) Asthma; brittle nails; bronchitis; colic (when the response to No. 8 Mag. Phos. is poor); dandruff; eczema; flashes of heat and chilliness; foul breath; gastric catarrh; giddiness of an inflammatory type; headache; intestinal catarrh; maintaining healthy hair; measles; menstrual disorders; minor skin eruptions with scaling or sticky exudation; palpitations; psoriasis; thick yellow mucous catarrh; third stage of inflammations; whooping cough; yellow coating of tongue.
- **No. 8 Mag. Phos.** (magnesium phosphate) Constipation; crampy labour pains, enlarged prostate; flatulence; gallstone colic; headache; hiccups; intercostal neuralgia; intermittent retention of urine and bladder spasm; kidney-stone colic; minor occasional pains; muscle cramps and spasms; neuralgia generally; ovarian neuralgia; painful menstruation; rheumatic pains; spasmodic shivers and twitching; stuttering; teething in infants; toothache when pains are sharp or shooting or boring; writer's cramp, and similar conditions.
- **No. 9 Nat. Mur.** (sodium chloride) Acne; anaemia (after seeing the doctor); asthma; chronic eczema; circulation problems; constipation (dry stools); diarrhoea; excessive salivation; excessive tears; gout; greasy skin; hayfever; headache (early morning); hysteria; influenza; insect bites and stings; loss of smell; loss of taste; minor haemorrhage; nettle rash; sciatica; shingles or herpes and blisters (with No. 1 Calc. Fluor.); shock; sneezing;

sterility; teething with excessive salivation; sunstroke; thin watery milk in lactation; ulceration of gums; water rash; watery colds with flow of tears and runny nose; watery vomiting.

- **No. 10 Nat. Phos.** (sodium phosphate) Acidity; all acid states of the bloodstream; acid taste; catarrh and thick yellow mucus; conjunctivitis; constipation; diarrhoea, gastric indigestion; giddiness; gout; grinding of teeth while sleeping; heartburn; incontinence from acidity; itching of nose; leucorrhoea; loss of appetite; morning sickness in pregnancy; nausea; red and blotchy face; rheumatic arthritis; rheumatism of joints; seasickness (with No. 6 Kali. Phos.); sick headache; sour breath; sour flatulence, sterility from acidity; to help prevent gallstones etc.; yellow-coated tongue.

- **No. 11 Nat. Sulph.** (sodium sulphate) Asthma of a watery nature; biliousness of a watery nature; bitter taste; bronchial catarrh; constipation; diarrhoea; digestive upsets; distended stomach; ear noises and earache from fluid retention; flatulence and colic; flu symptoms, gallbladder upsets; gout in watery subjects; hayfever; hydrocele (in the scrotum); kidney upsets; liver upsets; pancreatic upsets, queasiness; rheumatism 'in watery subjects'; to help with body water balance; tongue grey or greenish/brown; vomiting in pregnancy; warts.

- **No. 12 Silica** (silicon dioxide) Absent-mindedness; alcoholic intolerance; alopecia; asthma from dust; boils; brittle nails (in alternation with No. 7 Kali. Sulph.); chronic bronchitis; coccydynia; eyestrain; falling out of hair; fissures; foot sweats; ingrowing toenails; lack of stamina; pimples and spots; poor memory; premature ageing; styes; sweats, if unpleasant; whitlows.

There are also eighteen **combination remedies**, which are available from health-food shops and chemists. These bring together mineral salts that are known to be helpful with the same conditions and diseases.

The recommended doses of mineral salt remedies depend on the type and severity of the symptoms. Generally four tablets, three times a day, is the recommended dose for adults, but this can be increased if symptoms are severe. As the symptoms improve, the dose can be decreased. Usually the remedies should be taken until three days after the symptoms have ceased. The remedies are safe and it is impossible to overdose. Unlike other homoeopathic remedies, you can take the tablets at any time and do not have to give up coffee or tea. Tablets can be dissolved under the tongue; made up into a paste for external application, or added to boiled water or milk.

Tablets can be kept for up to three years once the bottle has been opened, provided that they are kept in a dry place away from sunlight.

Further reading

- Chapman, E. 1981. *About Biochemic Salts: essential micro-nutrients for health and vitality.* Wellingborough: Thorsons.
- Chapman, J. B. 1984. *Dr Schuessler's Biochemistry: a natural method of healing.* Wellingborough: Thorsons.
- Powell, E. F. W. 1977. *The Biochemic Prescriber.* Saffron Walden: C. W. Daniel.
- Schuessler, W. H. 1982. *Biochemic Handbook: how to get well and keep fit with the biochemic tissue-salts.* Wellingborough: Thorsons.
- Stanway, A. 1982. *A Guide to Biochemic Tissue Salts: a natural way to prevent and cure illness.* Redhill, Surrey: Van Dyke.

Bach flower remedies

Bach flower remedies are made from thirty-eight different species of wild flowers. They were developed in the 1930s by Dr Edward Bach, a homoeopath, doctor and bacteriologist, who selected them for the special abilities he believed they had. Bach argued that negative emotional states and personality problems were the cause of disease, and that these could be treated using particular flower remedies.

Dr Bach grouped his flower remedies into seven categories, according to the emotional state or personality type they could be used to treat:

- *'For those who have fear'* Aspen; Cherry Plum; Mimulus; Red Chestnut; Rock Rose.
- *'For those who suffer uncertainty'* Cerato; Gentian; Gorse; Hornbeam; Scleranthus; Wild Oat.
- *'For insufficient interest in present circumstances'* Chestnut Bud; Clematis; Honeysuckle; Mustard; Olive; White Chestnut; Wild Rose.
- *'For loneliness'* Heather; Impatiens; Water Violet.
- *'For those over-sensitive to influences and ideas'* Agrimony; Centaury; Holly; Walnut.
- *'For despondency and despair'* Crab Apple; Elm; Larch; Oak; Pine; Star of Bethlehem; Sweet Chestnut; Willow.
- *'For over-care for the welfare of others'* Beech; Chicory; Rock Water; Vervain; Vine.

As Julian Barnard explains in his book *A Guide to Bach Flower Remedies* (1987), 'Each category covers a range of mental and emotional states. Those concerned with fear, for instance, range from sheer terror (Rock Rose), to specific fears like a fear of heights or a fear of animals (Mimulus), to anxiety for the anticipated misfortunes of others (Red Chestnut)'.

The Bach flower remedies are prepared in two ways:

- *By 'the sunshine method'* A thin glass bowl is filled with pure water and the selected flowers are floated on the water, covering the surface. The bowl is then left in the sunlight for 3–4 hours (less if the blooms begin to fade). The healing energy Dr Bach believed to be contained within the flower is transferred into the water during this time. The flowers are then removed, and the liquid is poured into bottles with an equal volume of brandy (used as a preservative).
- *By 'the boiling method'* The selected parts of the plant are boiled in pure water for 30 minutes, then strained off and the liquid mixed with an equal volume of brandy.

Two drops of this extract or **essence** are then used to potentise a 30 ml (approximately) bottle of brandy. This becomes the **stock** of the remedy. To make up a prescription, 2 drops from between one and five stock remedies are put into 30 ml of water with a teaspoonful of brandy. The patient then takes 4 drops of this medicine four times a day for as long as required (usually for a few weeks).

Although there are some counsellors in Bach flower remedies, most people self-prescribe, as the remedies are very safe to use. Dr Bach discovered his remedies largely by intuition, and the use of the remedies relies heavily on an intuitive selection process. Some people select remedies by **dowsing**, using a pendulum which is held over each remedy in turn; prearranged signals for 'yes' and 'no' are noted each time the dowser 'asks' if a remedy is appropriate.

Research

According to Judy Howard, a consultant at The Dr Edward Bach Centre, and a qualified nurse, midwife and health visitor, 'There have been no clinical trials as such'. She says, however (personal communication 1993):

> The Bach remedies have been established now for nearly 60 years, and have gradually spread around the world from their humble beginnings to the present-day demands of worldwide distribution. All of this has occurred without any advertising campaign or active marketing involvement – the remedies have spread by word of mouth alone. Although this may not be quite the same as a structured clinical trial, the fact that the remedies have spoken for themselves in this way, is in itself evidence of their efficacy.
>
> We are constantly receiving good reports and results and there are many published case studies – *The Handbook of the Bach Flower Remedies* contains case studies on the use of each remedy, *Flower Remedies to the Rescue* offers case studies on the use of Rescue Remedy by lay people

and health professionals around the world, and we also publish some in the *Newsletter* which is issued three times each year.

Rescue Remedy is made from five of the thirty-eight Bach flowers, and can be taken in emergencies: for panic, shock, hysteria, mental numbness, and even unconsciousness. According to Christine Wildwood (1992), 'Although the Remedy cannot replace medical attention, it can alleviate much of the person's distress whilst they await the arrival of medical aid, thus enabling the bodymind's healing process to commence without delay.'

Recommended reading

- Bach, E. 1979. *The Twelve Healers and Other Remedies*. Saffron Walden: C. W. Daniel.
- Barnard, J. 1987. *A Guide to the Bach Flower Remedies*. Saffron Walden: C. W. Daniel.
- Chancellor, P. 1985. *Handbook of Bach Flower Remedies*. Saffron Walden: C. W. Daniel.
- Evans, J. 1985. *Introduction to the Benefits of the Bach Flower Remedies*. Saffron Walden: C. W. Daniel.
- Howard, J. n.d. *The Bach Flower Remedies Step by Step*. Saffron Walden: C. W. Daniel.
- Howard, J. n.d. *Bach Flower Remedies for Women*. Saffron Walden: C. W. Daniel.
- Vlamis, G. 1986. *Flower Remedies to the Rescue*. Wellingborough: Thorsons.
- Wildwood, C. 1992. *Flower Remedies*. Shaftesbury: Element Books.

Resources

Bach flower remedies

Bach Flower Remedies Ltd
Dr Bach Centre, Mount Vernon, Sotwell, Wallingford, Oxfordshire OX1 0PZ.

The Centre offers advice on the use of Bach flower remedies by post or by appointment. It also has register of counsellors in Bach flower remedies, and runs training courses and seminars.

References

- Barnard, J. 1987. *A Guide to Bach Flower Remedies*. Saffron Walden: C. W. Daniel.
- Dopson, L. 1988. An ailing alternative? *Nursing Times* **84**(48): 52–3.

- Gilbert, P. 1989. *Thorsons Complete Guide to Homoeopathically Prepared Mineral Tissue Salts*. Wellingborough: Thorsons.
- Hahnemann, S. 1810. *The Organon of Medicine*, reprinted 1983. London: Victor Gollancz.
- MORI/*The Times* 1989. Research, 21–5 August.
- NAHAT 1993. *Complementary Therapies in the NHS* (Research Paper No. 10). London: National Association of Health Authorities and Trusts.
- Stallick, J. 1990. Taking the lava cure. *Nursing Times* 86(28): 27–39.
- Swayne, J. 1992. The cost-effectiveness of homoeopathy: a pilot study and proposals for future research. *Homoeopathy* 42(5): 243–4.
- Swinnerton, T. 1990a. Alternative antenatal treatments. *Nursing Times* 86(48): 68–9.
- Swinnerton, T. 1990b. An alternative approach. *Nursing Times* 86(36): 66–7.
- Swinnerton, T. 1991a. Alternative postnatal therapies. *Nursing Times* 87(22): 64–5.
- Swinnerton, T. 1991b. Alternative remedies during labour. *Nursing Times* 87(9): 64–5.
- Wade, D. 1991. Is there a homoeopath in the house? *The Daily Telegraph*, November 23.
- Webb, P. 1992. *Homoeopathy for Midwives (& Pregnant Women)*. Available from the BHA.
- Wildwood, C. 1992. *Flower Remedies*. Shaftesbury: Element Books.
- Wolff, O. 1991. *Home Remedies: herbal and homoeopathic treatments for use at home*. Edinburgh: Floris Books.

11 HERBAL MEDICINE

Historical background

One thing that all races and people, past and present, have in common is the use of plants to treat the myriad of diseases and health problems that can beset us.

In the West, the origins of herbal medicine go back at least to ancient Egypt. Archaeologists have found papyri dating from 1550 BC which describe seven hundred plant medicines, many of which are still used today, and schools for herbalists are believed to have existed in ancient Egypt.

The ancient Greek physicians went on to add to the knowledge amassed by the Egyptians, having often been taught herbal medicine by Egyptian 'priest-doctors'. Of particular note are the Greek physicians Theophrastus and Dioscorides. Theophrastus (373–285 BC) is known as 'the father of botany' from his having written the *Historia Plantarum*, which became the standard textbook on botany for hundreds of years. It is also the oldest known Greek herbal. In the 1st century AD Dioscorides too wrote a seminal herbal, *De Materia Medica*. In it he brought together all that was then known about herbs, having had the opportunity to travel widely as a physician to the Roman armies of Emperors Claudius and Nero. Claudius Galen, who lived in the 1st and 2nd centuries AD, also compiled an important herbal, *De Simplicibus*; this, along with the Greek herbals, was much used by the Arab physicians of the 13th century.

The ancient Britons too knew their herbs. The woad with which they painted themselves before battle, for example, is now known to have had an antiseptic quality, which would have been helpful in the healing of any wounds soldiers received in battle. But little written knowledge from those times remains, although a thousand-year-old Saxon herbal, *The Leech Book of Bald*, is still in existence: this documents many herbs and herbal remedies.

During the so-called Dark Ages, knowledge of the medicinal properties of herbs was largely lost or confined to monasteries, and it was not until the Crusaders brought back information and books from the Arab world that herbal medicine was again used widely in Europe. For many years it was predominantly the monks who guarded this knowledge and who dispensed herbal remedies, made from herbs from their own gardens, to the sick. Once the printing press had been invented, however, herbal knowledge became accessible to anyone who could read, and its popularity spread – much to the alarm of the physicians of the day.

By the time of Henry VIII, physicians were sufficiently concerned to seek actively to protect their position. They managed to bring in legislation which would prevent a physician from practising unless he had first been 'examined by the Bishop of London or Dean of St Paul's calling to him four doctors physic'. The result was an acute shortage of physicians which led, in 1543, to Henry VIII reversing his original legislation in favour of a charter which allowed all his subjects to practise herbal medicine.

During the 16th and 17th centuries herbal medicine flourished, with the printing of many herbals. A few are still famous today, for example those of William Turner, John Gerard and Nicholas Culpeper.

But, by the 18th century, herbal medicine had begun to lose ground among physicians. Some have attributed this decline to herbalists' connections with astrology – the prescribing of plants according to the astrological sign to which they, and the disease to be treated, were attributed – and what were seen as rather unscientific beliefs such as the 'doctrine of signatures'. Put simply, this doctrine referred to the belief that the herb that would cure a particular disease would, in some way, look like the manifestations of the disease. So, for example, because the root tubers of the plant pilewort look a bit like haemorrhoids, they were used to treat this problem – quite successfully, as it happens; and pilewort is still used by some herbalists in treating this problem.

In reality, herbal medicine was a casualty of the new scientific age and the growth of a form of medicine which sought precise pharmacological remedies, not what were seen as unsavoury-looking whole-plant concoctions. The search for the 'active ingredients' of plants, the upsurge of pharmaceutical medicine and the age of the 'magic bullet' had begun, and the 'old ways' began to lose their potency.

Concerned by the plight of herbal medicine, herbalists banded together in 1864 to form the National Association of Medical Herbalists (now the National Institute of Medical Herbalists), which would register practitioners and standardise practice. Unfortunately, they still failed to get herbalists 'registered practitioner status' in the 1911 National Insurance Act.

Since then, like many other complementary therapies, herbal medicine has enjoyed a resurgence of interest; and in 1974 the World Health Organisation, in its World Health Directive, concluded that plant remedies could fulfil a need unmet by modern health-care systems. The WHO has gone on to encourage and support the efforts of developing countries to use plant remedies in an attempt to reduce their cash-strapped governments' expenditure on allopathic drugs.

In the late 1980s the first chair in herbal medicine was set up in France, at the University of Paris North, but it is still the case that only a tiny proportion of the money available for research worldwide is being used to investigate scientifically the efficacy of this, the oldest form of medicine known to humankind.

Further reading

- Boxer, A. & P. Black 1980. *The Herb Book*. London: Mayflower.
- Griggs, B. 1981. *Green Pharmacy*. London: Jill Norman & Hobhouse.

What is herbal medicine?

Herbal medicine refers to the use of plants in the promotion of healing and better health. While much modern allopathic medicine has its roots in plant remedies, herbal medicine differs in the way in which plants are used.

Whereas modern pharmacology seeks to identify and isolate the active ingredient in a plant – for example aspirin or other salicylates from willow bark, digoxin from foxglove, and quinine from cinchona bark – herbal medicine, known as the 'art of simpling', comprises remedies made from the whole plant or **simple**. Herbalists argue that the natural chemical balance present in a whole plant has a more holistic effect on the body than giving a patient just one active ingredient. There are also those who say that the unwanted side-effects of many drugs are the result of using the active ingredient 'out of context'. This is most obvious with Digitalis, Ipecac and Rauwolfia.

There are three basic principles to the art of simpling:

- Many diseases arise from the conditions created by the geography of the area in which they are found. Some herbalists believe that the same geographical features will produce plants that can be used to treat these diseases successfully.
- Only *mild* plants or herbs should be used in remedies, because these can be used freely and will have a gentle effect on the body.
- For some conditions, high doses of mild herbs and plants may be used in order to produce a required healing effect.

In the past, the time at which herbs were collected was seen as important. For example, many herbs were collected by moonlight, or when the dew was still on them. Remedies made from herbs collected in this way were thought to be more potent. Scientists have since found that, for example, the atropine content of Belladonna and the morphine content of Opium poppy juice can be four times greater in the early morning than at any other time.

Every herbal remedy is said to have three effects on the body: to detoxify it and to eliminate waste; to strengthen it and to help it heal itself; and to build up the organs.

Herbs can also be grouped according to which of the following effects they induce in the body:

- blood purification (made necessary because of problems such as air pollution and exhaustion) and neutralising the body's excess acidity;
- diuresis (balancing the body fluids);
- emesis (inducing vomiting);
- purging;
- stimulation (of the circulatory and/or nervous systems);
- sweating;
- tonification;
- tranquillisation.

Types of herbal remedies

A herbal remedy may be made from combinations of herbs or from a single herb. Remedies can be given to patients in several different ways. These include infusions, tinctures, oils, flower waters, and various other preparations.

Infusions

Typically 15 g of dried herb or root (or a handful of freshly chopped herb) and 575 ml of boiling water are mixed together and left for at least 10 minutes. Infusions are usually taken about 10–15 minutes before meals. Hard materials such as barks and roots are put in cold water, brought to the boil, and then simmered for 10–15 minutes, in order to make a stronger infusion called a **decoction**.

Tinctures

30 g of dried herb is mixed with 150 ml of appropriate-strength alcohol in a stoppered large glass jar; and then left for a month. The ingredients are stirred occasionally, making sure that the herb remains covered by the liquid. The liquid is then strained and the herb discarded. Usually a patient will take 5–10 drops three times a day, before meals. Children only need 1–5 drops three times a day, and babies 1 or 2 drops in milk or juice three times a day. (The dosage for adults may be increased to 15 drops, three times a day for three days, in serious cases.)

Oils

30 g of dried herb is mixed with 575 ml of oil (such as almond, sunflower or olive oil) in a glass bowl, and left covered in direct sunlight for 4–6 weeks. The bowl is then heated in a pan of hot water for 4–6 hours, and the liquid strained and bottled. The resultant oil can be made into creams or used as a massage oil. To make creams, 575 ml of herb oil is warmed and 3–4 tablespoons of lanolin or cocoa butter and 55 g of beeswax melted into it. The mixture is then beaten well and left to thicken into a creamy ointment. Tinctures in tiny quantities can be added to creams to increase their effect.

Flower waters

See Chapter 6, page 73.

Other preparations

These include tablets, poultices, suppositories, douches, enemas, smoking mixtures (herb blends), syrups, liniments, and salves.

Further reading

- Buchman, D. D. 1983. *Herbal Medicine: the natural way to get well and stay well*. London: Rider / The Herb Society.
- Christopher, J. R. 1976. *School of Natural Healing*. Published by the author.
- Hewlett-Parsons, J. 1981. *Herbs, Health and Healing*. Wellingborough: Thorsons.
- MacIntyre, M. 1988. *Herbal Medicine for Everyone*. London: Penguin.

Visiting a herbalist

A first appointment with a herbalist will usually last about an hour, during which time a detailed case history will be taken. Sometimes a physical examination may be necessary, for example measuring blood pressure or listening to the lungs.

The herbalist will be seeking to establish what is causing the symptoms, and to find a treatment that will restore the body's natural 'balance'. Any herbal remedies prescribed will usually be accompanied by a discussion of the patient's diet, level of exercise and lifestyle, with a view to making changes that may help with the problem under treatment. When prescribing herbal remedies, the herbalist will always take into account any allopathic drugs being taken. The Medicines Act 1968 enables a herbal practitioner to prescribe remedies 'in accordance with his own judgement as to the treatment required' after consultation and examination of the patient, so no one should expect to be treated by telephone.

After the initial consultation a patient's progress will be reviewed on subsequent visits and adjustments made to the herbal prescriptions if necessary.

The remedy prescribed will usually achieve its effect within three days, especially in acute cases. However, treatment should be continued for a week or two after the disappearance of symptoms to ensure a complete cure. For chronic conditions, a cure can take months. The general rule is that a month of treatment is needed for every year the condition has been suffered.

Indications

According to the National Institute of Medical Herbalists (see 'Resources'), 'The practice of herbal medicine offers the sufferer not just relief from symptoms but an improved standard of general health and vitality'.

For thousands of years people have been using herbs to treat many different health problems. Herbalists claim to be able to help most conditions, including those as disparate as allergies, heart and circulation problems, migraines, skin disorders, rheumatism and arthritis, menstrual disorders and respiratory infections.

With the growth in interest in herbal medicine, an increasing number of people are using herbal remedies as a form of self-help. Specialist herbal shops (see 'Resources') will give advice on the best herbs to use for particular conditions and how to prepare them; and prepared herbal remedies are now available for problems such as menstrual pain, insomnia and stress. Even large pharmacy chain stores have got in on the act with their 'own brands' of such remedies.

Some herbalists are unhappy about this trend: they argue that herbalism, like all complementary therapies, should be holistic in outlook, with each patient treated as an individual with special needs. A well-trained herbalist will not give herbal remedies to a patient without seeing him or her, as different remedies may be needed for patients suffering from the same complaint. Such a herbalist will treat each patient with an individualised remedy compounded from tinctures, plus an occasional external preparation. These practitioners generally agree that marketed products can lack the 'completeness' that they wish to give their patients, and that they need complementing with additional 'ingredients'.

However, for those who do want to use herbal remedies for simple ailments and conditions, there are many self-help herbal books on the market (see 'Recommended reading'). Two self-help remedies are reproduced in Box 11.1.

BOX 11.1
USEFUL HERBAL REMEDIES

Herbalist Elisabeth Brooke, in her book *Herbal Therapy for Women* (1992), offers a variety of simple, safe herbal remedies. For example, she suggests the following as a relaxing tea for headaches or insomnia:

- 14 g of Camomile flowers
- 14 g of Melissa flowers

Make the tea in the usual way, then allow it to stand for 10 minutes, covered. Sip slowly – sweetened, if really necessary, with just a little honey.

   For period pains, she suggests that 14 g of ginger root should be chopped and mixed with 14 g of yarrow. A tea is then made in the normal way, sweetened with honey and sipped slowly.

Contra-indications

Herbal medicines have an excellent safety record. Indeed, in the past twenty years licensed herbal medicines have received only ten 'yellow cards' (reports of adverse reactions, sent to the Committee on the Safety of Medicines).

   However, the Department of Health's Medicine Control Agency (MCA) has named the following herbs as having potential risks to health: Sassafras, Comfrey, Broom, Senecio Aureus, and Mistletoe. In addition, they say pregnant women should avoid Berberis, Black Cohosh, Blue Cohosh, Blood root, Fumaria, Helonias, Hydrastis, Juniper, Kelp, Mugwort, and Pennyroyal, as these may cause miscarriage in other than low doses. There are twelve more herbs whose use in practice is confined to the better-trained herbalists who know the risks and avoid them where appropriate.

   In the early 1980s Sassafras bark and its oil were withdrawn from licensed medicines because the oil, which constitutes 3–9 per cent of good bark, contains saffrole, a fragrant chemical which has shown carcinogenicity in rodents.

   When licensed medicines were reviewed by the MCA in 1988–90, Comfrey root was also withdrawn. Manufacturers of unlicensed tablets withdrew their products at the same time. The grounds were assumed liver toxicity and possible carcinogenicity, which has been proved for certain individual pyrrolizidine alkaloids in rodents. But such effects are still debatable for Comfrey itself.

   These herbal remedies failed the MCA's risk-benefit ratio assessment because the 'assumed' risks could not be balanced by positive evidence of benefit from clinical trial data – only qualitative statements of benefit were available, for example in the herbals. External preparations (such as ointments) containing Comfrey root are still licensed, as the alkaloids in question are not considered to be absorbed through intact skin.

In February 1993, the Ministry of Agriculture, Food and Fisheries (MAFF) publicised the decision by the Committee on Toxicity of Food (COT) that Comfrey root products sold as foods should be withdrawn. What is interesting, as Timothy Whittacker, chief chemist at Potter's (Herbal Supplies) Ltd points out, is that they did not object to the sale and use of Comfrey herb as a tea to be made by infusion or applied as a poultice. 'The decision recognised the widespread popular use of Comfrey in the country and sought to allow this to continue by not banning presentations of the herb which they know will yield low quantities of pyrrolizidine alkaloids on ingestion. Their publicity has sought to discourage the use of Comfrey leaves as a vegetable, and tablet or capsule forms of Comfrey herb which they perceive as concentrated presentations. Their somewhat political-looking decision took account of the presence of only four reports in the scientific literature of toxic events that might be associated with Comfrey consumption, alongside thousands of unharmed regular users.'

COT's review of Comfrey took fifteen months. COT now plans to look at Mistletoe, Broom, Life Root plant and Bearberry leaf. The timescale for each review is likely to be a year. If these too are withdrawn, another set of fairly widely used herbs will have been lost to us all despite having been prescribed by herbalists safely for centuries.

The debate over the safety of herbs and herbal remedies has been fierce and at times irrational. Herbs such as Comfrey and Sassafras bark have been banned from sale because, if taken in large quantities, they appear toxic in rats. However, we can still buy a packet of paracetamol over the counter, the contents of which – if taken at once – can kill. The public are, it seems, assumed to be sensible about allopathic drugs, but not about herbs.

The Eu expects any proprietary product to be the subject of a product licence if a medicinal claim is made, and it is encouraging the European Scientific Co-operation for Phytotherapy to produce more standard monographs for herbs. In the long term these will facilitate evaluation of herbs by government regulatory bodies, and perhaps prevent herbs being withdrawn unnecessarily.

Further reading

– Lust, J. 1983. *The Herb Book*. New York: Bantam.
– Pahlow, M. 1982. *Living Medicine: the healing properties of plants*. Wellingborough: Thorsons.

– Tobe, J. H. 1969. *Proven Herbal Remedies*. St Catherines, Ontario: Provoker.

Research

While specific herbal remedies have not generally been comprehensively investigated, the interest of allopathic medicine and the pharmaceutical industry in the medicinal properties of plants has led to research which has indirectly confirmed the appropriateness and efficacy of many old herbal remedies.

Evening Primrose

The Evening Primrose was used in poultices by the Native American Indians to heal bruises, its roots were brewed as a cough mixture, and the plant was also used for skin problems and asthma. In Europe too the plant was, for many years, known as 'King's Cure All'; combined with bramble tops, it was used as an ointment for getting rid of facial spots, while in Wales it was held that the juice was a cure for insanity.

According to Judy Graham (see below), herbals describe it as astringent and sedative. Evening Primrose oil is listed in such herbals as being helpful for gastro-intestinal disorders, asthma, whooping cough, female complaints, and wound healing. Yet it was not until the 1960s that research into the plant's medicinal properties was initiated. The oil from Evening Primrose seeds contains gammalinolenic acid (GLA), and has been found, for example, to be helpful in treating heart disease and vascular problems, rheumatoid arthritis, multiple sclerosis, schizophrenia, diabetes, hyperactivity in children, and eczema. Evening Primrose oil, in capsules, is now available on prescription for eczema and generalised breast pain. Evening Primrose oil is not, however, licensed as a remedy for any other conditions. There have been conflicting trial results in relation to the therapeutic value of Evening Primrose oil for pre-menstrual tension, although many women claim to have found it helpful.

For research references and more information on Evening Primrose oil, see:

– Graham, J. 1993. *Evening Primrose Oil*, revd edn. Wellingborough: Thorsons.

Feverfew

Feverfew is a member of the daisy family and has been used for hundreds of years as treatment for migraine. Johnson *et al.*'s double-blind placebo trial of the herb supported their hypothesis that Feverfew would reduce the frequency and severity of migraine attacks if taken prophylactically.

– Johnson, E. S., N. P. Cadam, & D. M. Hylands 1985. Efficacy of feverfew as a prophylactic treatment of migraine. *British Medical Journal* **291**(6495): 569–73.

Research methodology

As with many other complementary therapies, the question of how herbal medicine should be investigated has regularly been discussed. For a review of the issues see, for example:

– Mills, S. 1991. Herbal medicines: research strategies. *Complementary Medical Research* **5**(1): 29–35.

Other sources and examples of research

There are hundreds of research reports on individual herbs, and the list below is not meant to be comprehensive. For those keen to find out more about herbal research, there is a quarterly newsletter of research abstracts called *Greenfiles*. For more information and costs, write to:

Greenfiles
138 Oak Tree Lane, Mansfield NG18 3HR.

There is also a herbal database at the Centre for Complementary Health Studies at Exeter University.

The following list simply aims to illustrate the range of research now available.

– Adetumbi, M. A. & B. H. S. Lau 1983. *Allium sativum* (garlic) – a natural antibiotic. *Medical Hypotheses* **12**: 227–37.
– Chandler, R. F., *et al.* 1982. Ethnobotany and phytochemistry of yarrow. *Economic Botany* **36**(2): 203–23.
– Ernest, E. 1987. Cardiovascular effects of garlic: a review. *Pharmatherapeutica* **5**: 83–9.
– Fairburn, J. W. 1976. The anthraquinone laxatives. *Pharmacology* **14**, supplement 1: 7–101.
– Fintelmann, V. 1991. Modern phytotherapy and its uses in gastrointestinal conditions. *Planta Medica* **57**(7), supplement 1: 48–52.
– Holmes, F. A. 1991. Phase II trial of Taxol, an active drug in the treatment of metastic breast cancer. *Journal of the National Cancer Institute* **18**(83): 1797–1805.
– Houghton, P. J. 1988. The biological activity of valerian and related plants. *Journal of Ethnopharmacology* **22**: 121–42.
– Liu, C. X. 1992. Recent advances on ginseng research in China. *Journal of Ethnopharmacology* **36**(1): 27–38.
– Mills, S. 1991. Are herbs safe? *British Journal of Phytotherapy* **2**(2): 76–83.
– Savage, A. P. 1992. Adjuvant herbal treatment for gallstones. *British Journal of Surgery* **79**(2): 168.

The use of herbal remedies

Two nurses from Oregon in the USA conducted some interesting research into the use of herbal remedies by the general public: 100 adults were asked which of 50 listed herbs they or members of their families had used for health purposes, and with what effect. Of the 50, 22 were each used by 10 or more people; and all but 3 (Dock, White Ash and Pennyroyal) were used by at least 1 person.

– Brown, J. S. & S. A. Marcy,1991. The use of botanicals for health purposes by members of a prepaid health plan. *Research in Nursing and Health* 14(5): 339–50.

At the Centre for Complementary Health Studies at the University of Exeter, herbalist Simon Mills is currently developing the testing of therapeutic effects of herbal medicines in patients.

However, as Arthur Hollman, a consulting cardiologist at University College Hospital in London, explains in *Plants in Cardiology* (1992), of the 300 or so families of plant, only 22 are the source of major pharmaceutical drugs. He muses that 'There must be more plant medicines awaiting discovery, but how do we go about finding them?' How indeed, without a financial commitment to investigate the thousands of herbal remedies to be found in every country of the world?

Implications for nursing

Nurse tutor Jenni Frost has said (1992) that 'Nurses have a role to play in advising clients on the possible uses of herbal remedies, referring them to a qualified herbal practitioner if necessary'. If you agree with such an argument, it is important that you are competent to give such advice.

Quite rightly Ms Frost also warns, 'One of the great dangers of complementary therapies, however, is that people can become interested in one field and, rather than take an accepted training course (herbalism has a four-year training course to become a qualified practitioner), simply just become knowledgeable "dabblers". Such people may do more harm than good in their practice, certainly discrediting it in the eyes of medical professionals. Properly managed, herbal remedies can offer a safe and therapeutic complement to orthodox medication'.

Herbal medicine is not a therapy nurses can easily incorporate within their practice. There is no short cut to becoming a herbalist, and the UKCC is likely to take a dim view of a nurse who, without proper training or appropriate permission, has offered patients herbal remedies from the local health-food shop, even if she personally has found them helpful.

Resources

Herbal suppliers

G. Baldwin & Co.
173 Walworth Road, London SE17 1RW.

A mail-order service is available.

Neal's Yard
15 Neal's Yard, London WC2H 9DP.

A mail-order service is available.

Potter's (Herbal Supplies) Ltd (since 1812)
Leyland Mill Lane, Wigan, Lancashire WN1 2SB.

Some products are available by mail order.

Herbal remedies suppliers

When buying any remedy you should check the label to see whether it is a licensed medicinal product, controlled by the terms and conditions of its licence under the Medicines Act 1968. Currently there are fewer than five hundred licensed herbal products. A licensed product will carry two numbers on its label:

- the Product Licence number, 'PL......';
- the Manufacturer's Licence number, 'ML......'.

Such remedies have been produced under strict conditions and the ingredients have been controlled. The product will have had to satisfy a Department of Health assessor on the safety of the ingredients, the purity of the product (that is, that there are no contaminants), and the efficacy of the ingredients (proof that they do work). No such guarantees exist for unlicensed products. Tony Hampson is co-chairman of the Natural Medicines Group, director of the British Herbal Medicine Association (see 'Resources'), and managing director of Potter's; as he says, 'the PL or product licence should be regarded as the "MOT" of medicines'. Clearly there are reputable companies producing remedies that do not have a product licence but which are excellent, but it requires 'insider' knowledge to identify which companies they are.

The following companies produce a range of herbal remedies for a variety of conditions:

Gerard House (1965) Ltd
736 Christchurch Road, Bournemouth, Dorset BH7 6BZ.

D. Napier & Son Ltd
17–18 Bristo Place, Edinburgh EH1 1HA.

Potter's (Herbal Supplies) Ltd
Douglas Works, Leyland Mill Lane, Wigan, Lancashire WN1 2SB.

Frank Roberts (Herbal Dispensaries) Ltd
91 Newfoundland Road, Bristol BS2 9LT.

Weleda (UK) Ltd
Heanor Road, Ilkeston, Derbyshire DE7 8DR.

Leaflets on products from all of the above companies are available from the addresses given.

Training and regulation

The following organisations are involved in the training and regulation of herbalists:

National Institute of Medical Herbalists (NIMH)
9 Palace Gate, Exeter, Devon EX1 1JA.

The Institute was founded in 1864 and is the oldest body of practising medical herbalists. Membership is by examination, after completing a full-time course of training at the School of Herbal Medicine and a stipulated period of clinical practice. The Institute has a professional code of ethics and a disciplinary procedure. The Institute is also a member of the Council for Complementary and Alternative Medicine (see Chapter 1).

Those registered by the Institute can carry the letters MNIMH or FNIMH after their names. For a list of practitioners, write to the above address enclosing a large SAE.

School of Herbal Medicine (Phytotherapy) (SHM(P))
Bucksteep Manor, Bodle Street Green, nr Hailsham, East Sussex BN27 4RJ.

The NIMH and the School of Social Work and Health Sciences at Middlesex University have produced a four-year BSc honours degree course in herbal medicine. According to Brenda Cooke, the honorary treasurer, nurses have completed herbalist training at the School of Herbal Medicine.

General Council and Register of Consultant Herbalists (GCRCH)
Grosvenor House, 40 Sea Way, Middleton on Sea, West Sussex PO22 7SA.

The Council trains students by a correspondence course leading to an examination followed by a specified number of hours of practical clinical training. It also runs consulting rooms that operate under a code of ethics. Such practitioners may have MRH or FRH after their names.

There are other smaller training and registration bodies for herbalists, which claim to train to a level of competence appropriate for setting up a consultancy practice.

Useful addresses

British Herbal Medicine Association (BHMA)
P O Box 304, Bournemouth, Dorset BH7 6JZ.
or c/o Mr Ray Hill, Secretary and Code Administrator, Field House, Lye Hole Lane, Redhill, nr Bristol BS18 7TB.

The Association was established in 1964 'to combat the growing threat to the herbal industry inherent in the proposed Medicines Act legislation'. It helped ensure that the 1968 Act included special sections enshrining the right of herbal medicine to continue and for herbal remedies to be sold, other than through a pharmacy. The Association continues its dialogue with government to protect herbal medicine.

There is also a strong research element to the Association, and a commitment to 'do everything possible to advance the science and practice of herbal medicine and to further its recognition at all levels'. In this role it has produced the authoritative *British Herbal Pharmacopoeia* and the *British Herbal Compendium*. The pharmacopoeia was the result of a co-operative effort between senior experienced herbal practitioners and university personnel. It includes accurate descriptions and data setting standards for some 240 herbs, together with their therapeutic indications, products and dosage, and various other references of scientific interest.

Members of the Association include herbal practitioners, importers, manufacturers, wholesalers, herbal retailers, health-food shops, and users of herbal medicine, as well as some pharmacists, doctors and research workers in plant medicine.

Recommended reading

- Brooke, E. 1992. *Herbal Therapy for Women*. London: Thorsons.
- Ceres 1984. *The Healing Power of Herbal Teas*, Wellingborough: Thorsons.
- Culpeper, N. n.d. *Culpeper's Complete Herbal*. Slough: W. Foulsham.
- Gerard, J. 1975. *The Herbal*. London: Constable.
- Gosling, N. 1985. *Successful Herbal Remedies*. Wellingborough: Thorsons.
- Grieve, M. 1982. *A Modern Herbal*. London: Penguin.
- Griggs, B. 1981. *Green Pharmacy*. London: Jill Norman & Hobhouse.
- Griggs, B. 1982. *The Home Herbal*. London: Jill Norman & Hobhouse.
- Hewlett-Parsons, J. 1981. *Herbs, Health and Healing*. Wellingborough: Thorsons.
- Lust, J. 1983. *The Herb Book*. New York: Bantam.
- McIntyre, M. 1988. *Herbal Medicine for Everyone*. London: Penguin.
- Messeque, M. 1981. *Health Secrets of Plants and Herbs*. London: Pan.
- Mills, S. 1985 *The Dictionary of Modern Herbalism*. Wellingborough: Thorsons.
- Thomson, W. A. R. 1976. *Herbs that Heal*. London: A & C Black.
- Tiera, M. 1982. *The Way of Herbs*. San Francisco: Unity Press.

References

- Brooke, E. 1992. *Herbal Therapy for Women*. London: Thorsons.
- Hollman, A. 1992. *Plants in Cardiology*. London: British Medical Journal.
- Frost, J. 1993. Herbalism: an overview of an ancient art. *Professional Nurse* (January), 1: 237–41.

12 NATUROPATHY

Historical background

The term 'naturopathy' is fairly modern, having been coined in 1895 by John Scheel, a German doctor practising in the USA, to describe his particular methods of treatment, which involved hydrotherapy and 'hygienics'. Seven years later, Benedict Lust, who also practised in the States, applied this new word to a combination of natural therapies which aimed to 'raise the vitality of the patient to a proper standard of health'.

But the principles of naturopathy go back much further than that. The idea of a 'vital force' is common to many of the therapies discussed in other chapters, including those based on traditional Chinese medicine, but in the West it is the Hippocratic school of medicine, founded nearly two and a half thousand years ago, that probably laid the foundations of naturopathic thought.

Most folk medicine in Europe drew on the same principle of helping nature to get on with the job of healing, assisted by herbal medicines and changes of diet, but naturopathy as we know it today was formalised during the 19th century. 'Water cures' were becoming increasingly fashionable, and spa towns flourished; when railways were built, seaside towns would experience an unprecedented boom. In Bohemia, a man called Vincenz Priessnitz established something which sounds remarkably like a modern 'health farm' with its emphasis on pure water in large quantities, both internal and external, and lots of fresh air and exercises. Claims by Austrian physicians that he must be achieving such good results by other methods led to unsuccessful prosecutions and eventually an Imperial commission, the findings of which were so favourable that Priessnitz's business flourished.

In the 1850s, Claude Bernard, the French physiologist known as 'the father of experimental medicine', proposed a novel concept: *the milieu interieur*, or internal environment, whose stability was essential to health. This concept is more familiar to us nowadays as 'homoeostasis'. At about the same time, a German Dominican Father called Sebastian Kneipp was building on Priessnitz's work. His methods were espoused by founders of the health-farm movement in Britain; while Lust, mentioned earlier, was a Kneipp practitioner who in 1902 set up the American School of Naturopathy in New York.

In 1909 California was the first State to recognise naturopathy as a therapy, and its popularity grew until around the time of the Second World War, when advances in medical science seemed to offer faster, more effective treatments for bodily and mental ills. Interest steadily waned, but revived again during the 1960s, and has since gone from strength to strength.

In Britain, the British Naturopathic Association was founded in 1928, and the British College of Osteopathy and Naturopathy was established seven years later. A steady interest has been shown by the public ever since, although naturopathy has not had as high a public profile as some other therapies.

Further reading

– Inglis, B. 1979. *Natural Medicine*. London: Collins.

What is naturopathy?

'In watching disease, both in private houses and in public hospitals, the thing which strikes the experienced observer most forcibly is this, that the symptoms or the sufferings generally considered to be inevitable and incident to the disease are very often not symptoms of the disease at all, but of something quite different – of the want of fresh air, or of light, or of warmth, or of quiet, or of cleanliness, or of punctuality and care in the administration of diet, of each or all of these' (Nightingale 1860).

Florence Nightingale wrote these words in 1860, thirty-five years before the word 'naturopathy' was coined, yet they capture the essence of the therapy. **Naturopathy** – also known as **natural medicine, natural therapeutics**, and **natural cure** – is based on the principle that the body has an innate ability to heal itself. The postulated healing force is termed *vis medicatrix naturae*, 'the healing power of nature'.

What this means is that when the body is not functioning properly – when it is not 'healthy' – the best cure will be the one that comes from within, and the naturopath aims to help nature effect that cure. A strict interpretation of that principle would imply that naturopathic treatment should use nothing originating from outside the body, and there are certainly some practitioners who abide by that view, but many are trained in other disciplines, elements of which they may use in their practice.

Osteopathy and acupuncture, to give two examples of such other disciplines, are corrective measures which work by helping the person's innate tendency to health, and it could be argued that they are not introducing anything foreign to the body. The use of herbal and homoeopathic remedies might be more contentious, but, unlike orthodox medicine, the substances used are certainly 'natural'.

One thing on which all naturopaths are agreed is the idea that prevention is better than cure: naturopathy has long embodied all the elements of 'health promotion' which have been spelt out, in recent years, by practitioners of 'orthodox' medicine.

How it works

There are three underlying principles in naturopathy (Newman Turner 1990):

- the body will always strive towards equilibrium, or 'health';
- this equilibrium can be disturbed by the accumulation of toxins in the body;
- the body is its own best healer.

Symptoms, then, are a sign that the equilibrium has been disturbed, and there is no point in suppressing them. For example, if there is a raised body temperature, the naturopath would say that there is little value in giving a drug to bring the temperature down. (Orthodox medicine now holds that instead of being merely the result of increased metabolic activity as the immune system fights infection, higher than normal temperatures allow white blood cells to do their job more effectively – thereby bringing medical theory into line with that of naturopathy.) Instead, the aim of treatment is to establish the reason for the symptoms, and then to set about finding ways in which natural healing can take place, by ridding the body of toxins and accumulated waste products, and thereafter to ensure that the underlying cause does not recur. When the symptoms have gone, the person is not necessarily 'cured'; that can only be said to have happened when the body is in a fit enough state to make recurrence unlikely.

The naturopath, then, is not merely a therapist, in the sense of someone who makes a diagnosis and treats the condition; he or she is a teacher, too, who aims to help the person achieve an optimum state of health (as does the teacher of the Alexander technique – see Chapter 16).

Visiting a naturopath

Because so much of the treatment is related to lifestyle, a large part of the first consultation, which is unlikely to last for less than an hour, is dedicated to finding out as much as possible about the person and the way she or he lives and works. As so many disorders of the body can have an underlying psychological cause, a great deal of attention is paid to the mind.

In order to arrive at a diagnosis some naturopaths may order X-rays, blood tests and specialised scans like ultrasound or computerised tomography (CT).

If there is any indication that the patient has a problem which naturopathy alone cannot help, the practitioner will not hesitate to refer him or her to an appropriate physician.

Once the underlying problem has been identified, the practitioner will suggest changes in lifestyle that need to be made – changes which may be quite radical. Unsurprisingly, the first of these is likely to be dietary, because the innate healing forces within the body cannot function effectively if the person is not eating sensibly. This does not mean that a strict vegetarian diet will have to be followed, though: naturopathy treats the individual, not an idealised concept of how people should behave. The diet will be tailored to suit the person, and not the other way around.

In some cases, **fasting** may be necessary. There are several régimes, from a course of 3–5 days on nothing but water, to a restricted diet in which fruit juices and some vegetables might be allowed. The purpose of fasting is to give the body a rest, and to aid in detoxification.

It was mentioned earlier that many practitioners are trained in other disciplines, elements of which may be used in their treatment. Techniques which might be employed include the following:

- chiropractic or osteopathic manipulation;
- touch techniques, including massage, shiatsu, acupressure, and reflexology;
- acupuncture and traditional Chinese medicine;
- homoeopathy;
- yoga;
- physiotherapy;
- herbal medicine;
- hydrotherapy.

(Hydrotherapy – the therapeutic use of water in any form – has long been associated with naturopathy. In addition to the more familiar spa, sauna and sitz baths, it includes the use of douches, poultices, and colonic irrigation: Stanway 1987.)

The number of consultations necessary varies according to the person and the underlying problem or problems. Progress is monitored by the observation of three phenomena:

- Firstly, the general level of health rises steadily, punctuated by **healing crises**.

- Secondly, symptoms reappear, in the *reverse* order of their earlier appearance. This process may include symptoms which have previously been suppressed, but not fully resolved.
- Finally, the disease process moves from the inside outwards – that is, from deeper tissues towards the surface, and from vital organs to those that are less vital.

If the naturopath has been successful, once the original problem has been resolved, and provided that the patient maintains the lifestyle changes recommended by the practitioner, the probability of the problem recurring is significantly reduced.

Indications

Michael Murray and Joseph Pizzorno, in their *Encyclopaedia of Natural Medicine* (1990), give detailed recommendations about the naturopathic treatment – including preventive measures – of sixty-two specific conditions; these include skin problems, asthma, pre-menstrual syndrome, rheumatoid arthritis, AIDS, and dementia of the Alzheimer type.

For some conditions, particularly those involving the gastro-intestinal tract, the treatments are well tried, and few would argue with the sound physiological basis of the treatments and recommendations for changes in lifestyle (see Box 12.1); for others, though, more research is needed into the efficacy of naturopathy in their management (see 'Research').

BOX 12.1
AN EXAMPLE OF A NATUROPATHIC REMEDY

Problem: Cystitis

- *Recommended action* Cranberry juice, 450 ml per day; increase fluid intake to at least 3 litres per day.
- *General measures* Urinate after intercourse; restrict calories; avoid simple sugars and refined carbohydrates.
- *Nutritional supplements* Vitamin C, 500 mg 2-hourly.

(Adapted from Murray & Pizzorno 1990.)

This example shows that naturopathic remedies may, on occasion, mirror 'orthodox' treatment: increased fluid intake and acidification of the urine are the same measures that most conventional practitioners would advise for a bacterial infection of the urinary tract.

Contra-indications

As many practitioners say, people often come to them too late for effective treatment. A well-established acute infection is unlikely to respond to naturopathic treatment, but had the person consulted a naturopath earlier, it might never have manifested itself in the first place.

The use of fasting, while undoubtedly beneficial for many people, is potentially disastrous for others; in a Swedish study of 6 deaths and 27 admissions to intensive care that might have been the result of inappropriate 'alternative' therapies, the majority were related to fasting (Bostrom & Rossner 1990). This is not a problem that would arise with a properly trained naturopath, who would be well versed in nutrition, but anyone attempting self-treatment on 'naturopathic' lines runs some degree of risk.

Naturopathy has no place in the immediate treatment of medical/surgical emergencies or severe trauma: if the body's natural defences have been overwhelmed, practitioners of orthodox medicine have the necessary skills to intervene.

Research

Although individual elements of naturopathic treatment are well supported by research (for example, dietary elements of health, and the value of stress reduction), it is hard to find published reports of clinical studies of naturopathy. Roger Newman Turner, a leading British naturopath, has acknowledged this problem (1990): 'There is no doubt that the naturopathic profession has dragged its feet in assessing and recording its techniques'. While pointing out that the highly individualistic nature of the treatment makes controlled trials difficult to design, he goes on to say that 'a new research methodology needs to be devised'.

The Healing Aids Research Project

One small-scale trial, the Healing Aids Research Project (HARP), followed the progress of 16 HIV-positive patients who were treated along naturopathic lines for a year. Findings were presented by the researchers, L. J. Standish and J. Guiltinian, at an Arizonan conference in 1990; at the invitation of Lord Colwyn, they also presented their research in 1991 to the British Parliamentary Group on AIDS for further consideration.

The patients all received vitamin supplements and hydrotherapy, and when problems like diarrhoea and oral candidiasis (thrush) appeared, naturopathic remedies (homoeopathic or botanical) were used. At the end of the year, no subjects had gone on to develop full-blown AIDS, unlike comparable study groups in AZT trials, and subjective scores of well-being had improved in 12 out of 16 patients.

While uncontrolled, the trial seems to indicate that the role of naturopathic methods in the treatment of AIDS may be worth investigating further.

– Newman Turner, R. 1991. AIDS: signs of breakthrough. *Journal of Alternative and Complementary Medicine* (February), 12–13.
– Sofroniou, P. 1991. JACM presents seminar on AIDS. *NMS News* (October).

Implications for nursing

As the introduction suggests, the principles underpinning naturopathy would not have sounded odd to Florence Nightingale, and nearly 140 years later they do not jar with any more modern theories of nursing. The body *is* its own best healer; the best thing to do is help the body get on with it. As a partial definition of care, it has much to recommend it.

However, there are still misconceptions about naturopathy in some people's minds. If it were more widely discussed, many of those misconceptions could be corrected, and nurses could, perhaps, find much of value in the therapy. Without necessarily becoming practitioners, individuals might find that the application of naturopathic principles to the planning of care could have immense benefits for patients and clients.

Resources

Training and regulation

As with many therapies and disciplines, anyone can call him- or herself a naturopath. However, the chief professional and regulatory body is the General Council and Register of Naturopaths.

British Naturopathic Association (BNA)
Frazer House, 6 Netherhall Gardens, London NW3 5RR.

Established in 1928, the BNA maintains the General Council and Register of Naturopaths. A copy of the Register of members can be obtained from the Association for a small fee.

Training in naturopathy takes four years, full-time, and leads to the award of BSc (Honours). Anatomy, physiology and pathology take up a large part of the curriculum. Further details can be obtained from:

British College of Naturopathy and Osteopathy
Frazer House, 6 Netherhall Gardens, London NW3 5RR.

Graduates of this college may use the letters ND (Naturopathic Diploma) after their names, and use the title 'Registered Naturopath'. 'MRN' signifies membership of the Register.

Recommended reading

- Campbell, A. (ed.) 1984. *Natural Health Handbook*, reissued 1991. London: Burlington.
- Murray, M. & J. Pizzorno 1990. *Encyclopaedia of Natural Medicine*. London: Macdonald Optima.
- Newman Turner, R. 1990. *Naturopathic Medicine: treating the whole person*, revd edn. Wellingborough: Thorsons.
- Stanway, A. (ed.) 1987. *The Natural Family Doctor: hydrotherapy*. London: Gaia.

References

- Bostrom, H. & S. Rossner 1990. Quality of alternative medicine – complications and avoidable deaths. *Quality Assurance in Health Care* 2(2): 111–17.
- Murray, M. & J. Pizzorno 1990. *Encyclopaedia of Natural Medicine*. London: Macdonald Optima.
- Newman Turner, R. 1990. *Naturopathic Medicine: treating the whole person*, revd edn. Wellingborough: Thorsons.
- Nightingale, F. 1860. *Notes on Nursing: what it is, and what it is not*, reprinted 1980. Edinburgh: Churchill Livingstone.
- Stanway, A. (ed.) 1987. *The Natural Family Doctor: hydrotherapy*. London: Gaia.

13 ACUPUNCTURE

Historical background

Some time – as far back as 7000 years ago, so one story goes – Chinese physicians observed that soldiers wounded by arrows sometimes recovered from illnesses, unrelated to their injuries, which had afflicted them for many years. From such an event, it has been suggested, the Chinese developed the principle of acupuncture: that many diseases and conditions can be treated by penetrating the skin at particular points. Presumably the Chinese went on to establish that the size of the wound did not matter, only its exact location. And that the effects of the arrow could be reproduced by artificially puncturing the skin.

The truth of this story is debatable, but it serves to illustrate the basis of acupuncture, and indeed of traditional Chinese medicine generally: the importance of detailed observation.

Whatever acupuncture's actual origin, it is thought that needles were first made of stone, then from wood, bones and ceramic. Bronze needles began to replace the others at the time of the Chang dynasty, around 3000 years ago. Nowadays needles are usually made of stainless steel.

At first it was thought that different metals had different effects. For example, the Chinese believed that a gold needle acted to stimulate, and silver to sedate. In China this approach fell into disuse, physicians concentrating instead on the mode of application of the needles in order to produce the effect they required. In Japan, however, acupuncturists still adhere to the principle that needles made from different metals have different effects.

By the process of detailed observation, Chinese physicians identified which points on the skin affected and controlled which organs, and went on to show that by penetrating such points with needles, a wide range of diseases could be cured.

The earliest writings on acupuncture date back 4500 years, to when thirty-four books were published under the title *Nei Jing*. This collection took more than 1500 years to complete, and the wisdom it contains still forms the basis of traditional Chinese medicine today, underpinning the use of herbs (see page 185), acupuncture, diet, manipulation, massage, hydrotherapy, sun and air therapy, and exercise.

The earliest extant work devoted exclusively to acupuncture and moxibustion (applying heat from burning herbs to acupuncture points) is *A Classic of Acupuncture and Moxibustion*, published in AD 259. In this book, the name and the number of points of each channel and their exact locations are defined and systemised, and the properties and indications of each point and the methods of needling described.

During the 7th century AD the use of acupuncture spread to other Far Eastern countries, including Japan, and acupuncture continued to flourish as a form of treatment well into the 20th century.

There was a temporary decline in its popularity during the late 19th and early 20th centuries, as Western medicine was introduced into China. Indeed in 1914 and 1929 the Chinese government tried to ban all forms of traditional Chinese medicine. But its roots were too deep, and after the People's Republic of China was created in 1949, studies were initiated to investigate the efficacy of traditional Chinese medicine. Hundreds of papers reporting experiments and clinical trials were published, and on the basis of their findings, traditional and modern medicine were accorded equal status in the health-care system.

Even today, modern and traditional medicine coexist in China's health-care system, to the extent that since 1958 more than one million operations have been performed using needles instead of chemical anaesthesia. Currently there are around a half a million acupuncturists practising in China.

Acupuncture was brought to the West in the last century by Jesuit missionaries who had travelled in China and the East. In Europe there are now over five thousand acupuncturists, and the value and efficacy of acupuncture in treating a wide range of conditions is accepted in most countries in the world.

Further reading

– Beau, G. 1972. *Chinese Medicine*. New York: Avon.
– Duke, M. 1973. *Acupuncture*. London: Constable.

What is acupuncture?

The International Register of Oriental Medicine (see 'Resources') describes **acupuncture** as 'a system of medicine which restores and maintains health by the insertion of fine needles into specific points on the surface of the body. The action of needling these points stimulates the body to rebalance itself, catalysing homoeostasis by activating our own recuperative and self-healing powers'. Most acupuncturists would agree that this definition encapsulates the main principles of acupuncture.

Traditional Chinese medicine and acupuncture have developed from a very different philosophical system to that practised in the West. Medicine here is rooted in our scientific tradition of seeking the cause of an event and developing scientific laws to explain why the event happens as it does. Such an approach arises in part from the predominant religious belief system in the West – that of a 'creator' God.

In contrast, the Chinese emphasise the importance of order and pattern. For them, there is no creator God, only the 'seamless web' of the universe, a web that has no weaver. Truth is there for everyone with eyes to see; wisdom and knowledge come by attuning oneself ever more finely to the rhythm of the universe – the **Tao**, or 'Way or Life'. According to traditional Chinese medicine, to live in harmony with the Tao is essential if people are to realise their full potential during their lifetime. The Chinese believe that in order to live more in tune with the Tao, we need to ensure that our lives are in balance – activity balanced with rest, excitement with reflection, and so on.

How it works

At the level of the individual, the Chinese believe there are three aspects to a person's being, the **Three Treasures**:

- **Jing** The deep or 'reserve' energy that sustains us. The Jing is the basic power structure of the body which determines an individual's sexual, mental, and defensive energies.
- **Qi** The life force or 'vital' energy of the body.
- **Shen** The spirit energy which relates to an individual's attitude, consciousness, and mind.

Qi is central to acupuncture theory and is fundamental to traditional Chinese medicine. Acupuncturist Wainwright Churchill (1988) explains it thus: 'Every aspect of the human body pertains to different types of Qi with different qualities and functions. The organs have particular functions and generate or affect various types of Qi. In health, the different types of Qi of the body interact harmoniously, producing wellbeing on all levels – physical, emotional, psychological and spiritual. In illness, specific types of Qi may be deficient or in excess, producing imbalances which manifest as feeling unhealthy, and leading to symptoms which might be physical, emotional, psychological or indeed, spiritual'.

An acupuncturist seeks to understand the nature of the patient's Qi in order to establish how best to use his or her skill to bring the patient back to a more harmonious state of health.

According to the Chinese, Qi flows through the body in channels called **Meridians** (Figure 13.1a–c). There are twelve 'main' Meridians which are associated with major **Organs**, although two of

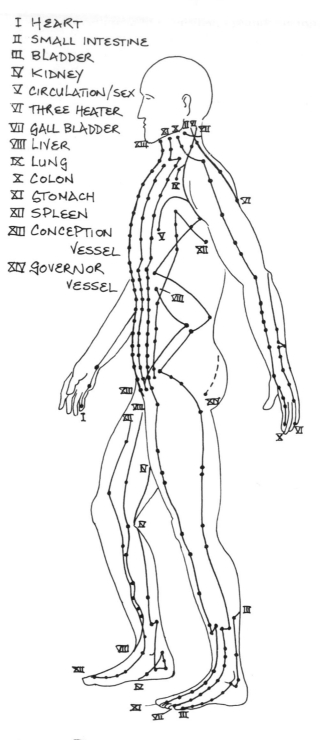

I HEART
II SMALL INTESTINE
III BLADDER
IV KIDNEY
V CIRCULATION/SEX
VI THREE HEATER
VII GALL BLADDER
VIII LIVER
IX LUNG
X COLON
XI STOMACH
XII SPLEEN
XIII CONCEPTION VESSEL
XIV GOVERNOR VESSEL

FIG 13.1(a): THE MERIDIANS OF QI ENERGY (SIDE VIEW)

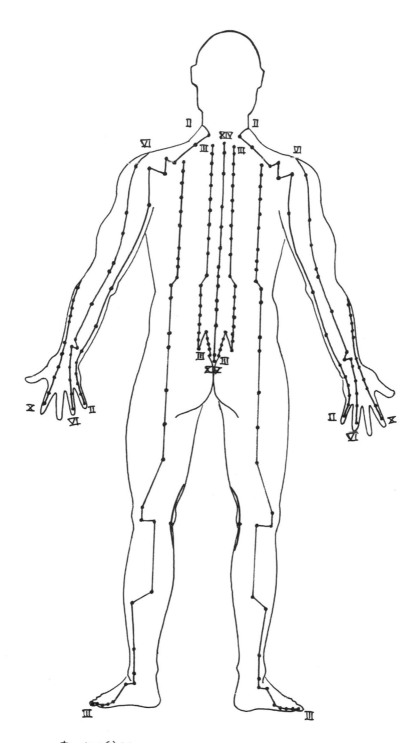

fig 13.1(b) MERIDIANS OF QI ENERGY (REAR VIEW)

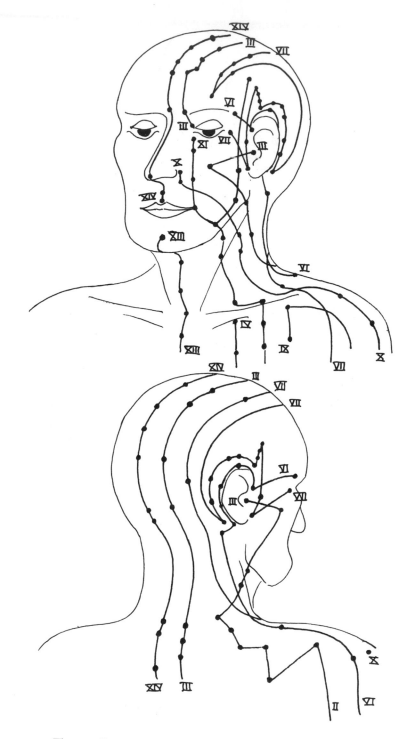

Fig 13.1 (c) MERIDIANS OF QI ENERGY (HEAD & NECK)

these 'Organs' – the Pericardium and Triple Heater – are not organs in the Western meaning of the word. In traditional Chinese medicine an Organ is defined by its *function*, not its structure or location. Organs have a much wider range of functions attributed to them: physical, psychological, emotional and spiritual. Moreover, if an organ is removed, the functioning of the Meridian still continues.

Along each Meridian there are the **points**. Each point has a particular influence on the Qi. An acupuncturist inserts a needle into a specific point in order to influence the Qi in a particular way.

In additional to the twelve main Meridians there are eight 'extraordinary' Meridians, of which two have their own points. The others share points that are to be found on the twelve main Meridians. Other Meridians also exist which are associated with the twelve main Meridians.

When treating disease, an acupuncturist tends to think in terms of the **depth** of illness. More superficial illnesses will relate to a problem in a particular Meridian, whereas more profound illness relate to the Organ itself. However, acupuncturists consider that if a superficial illness is not treated, eventually there will be an effect on the Organ.

Two other concepts are important in gaining an understanding of acupuncture – Yin/Yang and the Five Elements.

Yin and Yang

Originally **Yin** meant 'the shady side of the slope or the north bank of a river'; and **Yang** meant 'the sunny side of a slope or the south bank of a river'. These meanings were later extended to express the delicate balance of dark (Yin) and light (Yang). As Mole (1992) explains, 'Yin and Yang are not substances, but are an expression of the two poles of fundamental duality that exists in nature'. This balance embraces all opposites: female and male, cold and heat, passivity and activity, repose and motion. The black and white dots indicate the flow of one aspect into another (Figure 13.2).

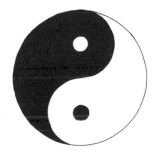

Fig 13.2: Yin & Yang symbol

The relationship between Yin and Yang is dynamic: Yin is always transforming itself into Yang, and vice versa. Ideally there is an equilibrium, but if the harmony is lost, disease results.

In making a diagnosis, an acupuncturist assesses the patient's Qi and the relationship between his or her Yin and Yang nature. In particular, the acupuncturist will try to assess the level of balance between the following 'opposites' in the patient:

Yang	Yin
Fire	Water
Heat	Cold
Dry	Wet
Hyperactive	Hypoactive

When these opposites are out of balance, the health of an individual is compromised. For example, fire represents the flame that maintains the body's metabolism, and water moistens and calls the body's physiological functions. When there is too much water, it will excessively dampen the fire, thus undermining the body's metabolism.

The Five Elements

The concept of the **Five Elements** (Figure 13.3) is probably not as old as that of Yin/Yang, but still dates back some three thousand years.

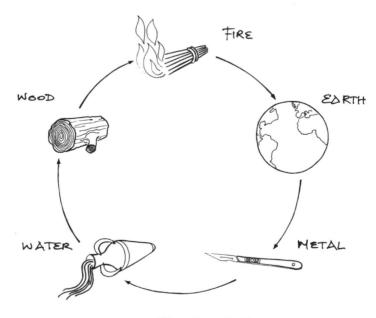

FIG 13.3 : THE FIVE ELEMENTS

The five Elements are **Water, Metal, Wood, Fire** and **Earth**. Each is associated with a season, certain emotions and particular Organs:

Element	Season	Emotion	Organs
Wood	Spring	Anger	Liver; Gallbladder
Fire	Summer	Joy	Heart; Small Intestine; Heart Protector; Triple Heater
Earth	Late summer	Pensiveness/ Obsessiveness	Spleen; Stomach
Metal	Autumn	Grief	Lungs; Large Intestine
Water	Winter	Fear	Kidney; Bladder

Each Element also represents a different quality in a person, in the same way as the seasons each bring a different quality to the natural world.

The Five Elements interact and influence each other and are often depicted in a circle. Any imbalance in one Element disturbs the whole cycle and affects the Qi.

What causes disease?

In Chinese medicine the body, mind and spirit are inextricably linked. The causes of disease can, in Chinese terms, be either *external* (that is, climatic), in which case they affect the body; or *internal* (that is, emotional), in which case they affect the mind and the spirit first. The Chinese believe that external causes of disease will only affect an individual whose Qi is already compromised in some way. Such external causes include wind, heat, cold, damp, dryness, diet, and levels of sexual activity (the Chinese are firm believers that too much sex is bad for you). Internal causes of disease relate to the effect extremes or excesses of particular emotions – anger, joy, worry or pensiveness, grief, fear, and fright – can have on a person's health.

In all things, the Chinese advocate following **the middle way**, avoiding extremes in order to promote health, happiness and longevity.

Diagnosis

To make a diagnosis, an acupuncturist uses a variety of methods. In addition to asking the patient about his or her health – past and present – and observing how the patient looks and acts, an acupuncturist will also inspect the patient's *tongue* and palpate the wrist *pulse*.

When looking at the tongue, the acupuncturist will note its colour, shape and coating. Different areas of the tongue are associated with particular Organs, and will give the acupuncturist information on the state of health of those Organs. In Chinese medicine there are twenty-eight qualities attributed to the pulse, which can be felt for in six different wrist positions, using three fingers. The acupuncturist will note the quality and relative strength of each. As Churchill (1988) notes, 'a good acupuncturist may often startle a patient with insights from these two examinations, for example, by noting that a person has had a glass of wine in the past week'.

An acupuncturist will also ask the patient to describe any symptoms, which may also help establish which Organs are affected.

Treatment

An acupuncturist will always consider the patient's presenting *symptoms* and the deep *causes* of the problem alongside each other. Profound treatment will always seek to get to the cause of the problem.

There are essentially three treatment alternatives open to an acupuncturist:

- clear the symptoms, then treat the causes;
- treat the two simultaneously; or
- treat the cause, in which case the symptoms will automatically clear up.

Which route a given practitioner takes is largely a matter of personal style.

Visiting an acupuncturist

A first appointment will usually take between an hour and an hour and a half. The acupuncturist will take a detailed case history, feel the patient's pulse and look at his or her tongue.

Treatment primarily involves the insertion of very fine needles into specific points on the surface of the body. How many needles are used and where they are placed will depend on the diagnosis.

The needles used are very fine and are inserted very lightly – generally only a little way into the skin. Patients report feeling a tingling sensation at the point where the needle is inserted: this is known as the **De Qi**, and indicates that the needle has been inserted in the correct location. The process is generally not painful. The needles will be left in anything from ten minutes to an hour. All needles used are sterilised, and, since the advent of AIDS, many acupuncturists now use disposable needles.

Other forms of treatment which the acupuncturist may use include warming the points by burning a dried herb called **moxa** over them; **acupressure**, which is especially effective for children; or stimulating points with a mild electrical current. Additionally the **plum-blossom needle** may be used: this has a two-sided head, on each of which are fine spikes which are used to stimulate an area rather than a point. An acupuncturist will also make suggestions about lifestyle changes that may help improve the condition and aid healing.

After treatment, patients have reported feeling relaxed, elated, or 'walking on air'. Occasionally a patient may feel worse before feeling better.

The number of treatments necessary will depend on the problem – chronic conditions will take longer to treat than acute illness.

Indications

In the West, acupuncture is associated primarily with relieving pain and helping with addiction problems, although most people are also aware that the Chinese use acupuncture as a form of anaesthetic.

In fact, there are few conditions that acupuncture has not at some point been used to treat. Even the World Health Organisation has compiled a provisional list of diseases and conditions for which they consider treatment with acupuncture to be appropriate. This includes the following:

- *Respiratory system* Acute bronchitis and bronchial asthma.

- *Upper respiratory tract* Acute sinusitis; acute rhinitis; common cold; acute tonsillitis.

- *Gastro-intestinal system* Spasms of oesophagus and cardia; hiccup; acute and chronic gastritis; gastric hyperacidity; chronic duodenal ulcer (pain relief); acute duodenal ulcer (without complications); acute bacillary dysentery; constipation; diarrhoea; paralytic ileus.

- *Disorders of the mouth* Toothache; post-extraction pain; gingivitis; acute and chronic pharyngitis.

- *Disorders of the eye* Acute conjunctivitis; central retinitis; myopia (in children); cataract (without complications).

- *Neurological and musculoskeletal disorders* Headache; migraine; trigeminal neuralgia; facial palsy (early stage); pareses following a stroke; peripheral neuropathies; sequelae of poliomyelitis (early state); Meniere's disease; neurogenic bladder dysfunction; nocturnal enuresis; intercostal neuralgia; cervicobrachial syndrome; 'frozen shoulder'; 'tennis elbow'; sciatica; low back pain; osteoarthritis.

Acupuncturists in this country and abroad would argue that the list of conditions they commonly treat is much wider. In addition to those recognised by the WHO, acupuncture is also used to treat conditions as wide-ranging as gynaecological problems; problems during pregnancy and childbirth; addictions; impotence in men; urinary problems; insomnia; schizophrenia; varicose veins; vertigo; eczema; colitis; infectious hepatitis; and shingles.

Traditionally, acupuncture has been used to maintain health. In China, many people still book an appointment with an acupuncturist at the turn of each season to maintain good health. In the past, acupuncturists in China were paid only while their patients remained healthy. Indeed one of the most famous passages in the *Nei Jing* (see 'Historical background') argues that, 'When medicinal therapy is initiated only after someone has fallen ill, when there is an attempt to restore order only after unrest has broken out, it is as though someone has waited to dig a well until he is already weak from thirst, or as if someone begins to forge a spear when the battle is already under way. Is this not too late?'

According to the British Acupuncture Association (see 'Resources'), 'Acupuncture is not a panacea and should be combined with other therapies for the treatment of degenerative illnesses. It can be said that acupuncture can usefully treat every condition but not cure every individual case'.

Contra-indications

Some diseases (mainly wasting diseases) are difficult to cure with acupuncture if they have progressed to a point where the body has become very thin. As acupuncture works by restoring an energetic balance to the body and stimulating its own healing powers, if the body is depleted there are no reserves to call on and healing is very slow.

Research

There has been an enormous amount of research into acupuncture, much of it concentrating on its efficacy as a method of pain relief; only a selection is reproduced below. There are, however, useful review articles and books which have brought together some of the classic pieces of research, including the following:

- Bensoussan, A. 1990. *The Vital Meridian*. Edinburgh: Churchill Livingstone.
- Vincent, C. A. & P. H. Richardson 1986. The evaluation of therapeutic acupuncture concepts and methods. *Pain* **24**: 1–13.

- Vincent, C. A. & P. H. Richardson 1987. Acupuncture for some common disorders: a review of evaluative research. *Journal of the Royal College of General Practitioners* **37**: 77–81.
- Xiangtong, Z. (ed.) 1986. *Research on Acupuncture, Moxibustion and Acupuncture Anaesthesia*, trans. H. T. Chang. Beijing: Science Press (Berlin: Springer Verlag).

There is also a wide range of articles which discuss the methodology that should be used to investigate acupuncture, such as these:

- Bensoussan, A. 1991. Contemporary acupuncture research: difficulties of research across scientific paradigms. *American Journal of Acupuncture* **19**(4): 357–65.
- Lewith, G. T. 1984. Can we assess the effects of acupuncture? *British Medical Journal* **288**: 1475–6.
- Vincent, C. A. 1990. Credibility assessment in trials of acupuncture. *Complementary Medical Research* **4**(1): 8–11.
- Vincent, C. A. 1992. Acupuncture research: why do it? *Complementary Medical Research* **6**(1): 21–4.
- Vincent, C. A. & P. Mole 1989. Acupuncturists and research. *Complementary Medical Research* **3**(3): 25–30.
- Vincent, C. A. & P. H. Richardson 1986. The evaluation of therapeutic acupuncture: concepts and methods. *Pain* **24**: 1–13.
- Watson, K. B. 1991. The philosophical basis of traditional Chinese medicine and the implications for its clinical evaluation. *Journal of Chinese Medicine* **36**: 14–17.

Studies which have looked at the efficacy of acupuncture in the treatment of particular problems include:

- Boxx, P. J. 1984. Acupuncture in childbirth. *British Journal of Acupuncture* **7**: 22–4.
- Bullock, M. L. 1984. Controlled trial of acupuncture for severe recidivist alcoholism. *Lancet* **i**: 1435–9.
- Diankui, G. 1986. Efficacy of acupuncturing the Jianjing point in 393 cases of acute mastitis. *Journal of Traditional Chinese Medicine* **6**: 1–20.
- Dickens, W. & G. T. Lewith 1989. A single-blind, controlled and randomised clinical trial to evaluate the effect of acupuncture in the treatment of trapezio-metacarpal osteoarthritis. *Complementary Medical Research* **3**(2): 5–8.
- Dundee, J. W., W. N. Chestnutt & R. G. Ghaly 1986. Traditional Chinese acupuncture: a potentially useful antiemetic? *British Medical Journal* **293**(6): 583–4.
- Ellis, N., *et al.* 1990. The effect of acupuncture on nocturnal urinary frequency and incontinence in the elderly. *Complementary Medical Research* **4**(1): 16–17.
- Gaw, A. C., L. W. Chang & L. C. Shaw 1975. Efficacy of acupuncture on osteoarthritic pain. *New England Journal of Medicine* **293**: 375–8.
- Gunn, C. C., W. E. Milbrandt, A. S. Little & K. E. Mason 1980. Dry needling of muscle motor points for chronic low-back pain: a randomized clinical trial with long-term follow-up. *Spine* **5**: 279–91.

- Jio, X., X. Chang, K. Yin, & Y. Gao 1992. Clinical and experimental studies on acupuncture therapy of stroke-related blood stasis. *International Journal of Clinical Acupuncture* **3**(3): 229–41.
- Jobst, K. 1986. Controlled trial of acupuncture for disabling breathlessness. *Lancet* **ii**: 1416–18.
- Junnila, S. Y. T. 1982a. Acupuncture superior to piroxicam in the treatment of osteoarthritis. *American Journal of Acupuncture* **10**: 241–6.
- Junnila, S. Y. T. 1982b. Acupuncture therapy for chronic pain: a randomised comparison between acupuncture and pseudo-acupuncture with minimal peripheral stimulus. *American Journal of Acupuncture* **10**: 259–62.
- Lewith, G. T. 1984. How effective is acupuncture in the management of pain? *Journal of the Royal College of General Practitioners* **34**: 275–8.
- Macpherson, H. 1992. The treatment of neck and upper back pain with acupuncture. *Journal of Clinical Medicine* (February), **38**: 22–6.
- Marcus, P. 1990. Integration of acupuncture within a pain relief clinic. *Acupuncture in Medicine* **19**(4): 305–13.
- Mendelson, G., T. S. Selwood, H. Kranz, *et al.* 1983. Acupuncture treatment for chronic back pain: a double-blind placebo-controlled trial. *American Journal of Medicine* **74**: 49–55.
- Rempp, C. 1991. Pregnancy and acupuncture from conception to postpartum. *American Journal of Acupuncture* **19**(4): 305–13.
- Richardson, P. H. & C. A. Vincent 1986. Acupuncture for the treatment of pain: a review of evaluative research. *Pain* **24**: 15–40.
- Ter Riet, G., J. Kleijnen & P. Knipschild 1990. A meta-analysis of studies into the effect of acupuncture on addiction. *British Journal of General Practice* **40**(338): 379–82.
- Vincent, C. A. 1990. A controlled trial of the treatment of migraine by acupuncture. *The Clinical Journal of Pain* **5**: 305–12.
- Weintraub, M., S. Petursson, M. Schwartz, *et al.* 1975. Acupuncture in musculo-skeletal pain. Methodology and results in a double-blind controlled trial. *Clinical Pharmacology and Therapeutics* **17**: 248.
- Ziaoma, W. 1987. Observations on the therapeutic effects of acupuncture and moxibustion in 100 cases of dysmenorrhoea. *Journal of Traditional Chinese Medicine* **7**: 31.

Attempts to explain how acupuncture works generally fall into three main categories: those that argue that the nerve fibres carry and transmit the acupuncture effect (see, for example, Lu *et al.* 1981; Melzack 1978); those that argue that the acupuncture effect is via the circulation of neurotransmitters and other hormones in the cerebrospinal fluid and in the bloodstream, in particular endorphins (see, for example, Mayer *et al.* 1977; Zhang *et al.* 1980; Price & Rees 1982; Darras *et al.* 1992); and those that argue that the Meridians are electrically distinct and that changes within them are responsible for triggering the neural and humoral responses (see, for example, Becker 1974; Jessel-Kenyon *et al.* 1992). However, no Western scientific theory has proved wholly satisfactory in explaining how acupuncture works.

Implications for nursing

The Council for Acupuncture (see 'Resources') states that: 'It is essential that only properly qualified practitioners should treat people with acupuncture, because it takes several years of training in acupuncture to understand the changes in energy that cause symptoms to appear'. Nurses should not contemplate the use of acupuncture with patients unless they have received appropriate training. However, there is considerable debate about what consti tutes an 'appropriate training'.

There are medically qualified doctors and some nurses treating patients with acupuncture. Many belong to The British Medical Acupuncture Society (see 'Resources'), which currently has over six hundred members. While some have undergone rigorous train-ing, others may have attended only a few weekend courses. Yet the BMAS believes that acupuncture 'should be practised as a branch of medicine' and they recommend that potential patients should 'go to a fully registered medical practitioner who is trained and experienced in acupuncture'. The BMAS gives three reasons for this advice:

- A qualified doctor has been trained to discover whether a patient has a condition requiring other urgent medical treatment. He or she will not hesitate to advise a patient if acupuncture does not seem suitable.
- You can be sure that a qualified doctor has the necessary anatomical training and will follow the correct hygiene proce-dures with sterile needles, to eliminate the risk of transmitting infections such as AIDS or hepatitis.
- A medical practitioner will be able to communicate with other doctors, such as the patient's GP, or any hospital specialists who may also have been consulted. He or she will be able to gain access to medical records or X-rays and can order further investi-gations if these are indicated.

In fact, non-medically-qualified acupuncturists whose names appear on the Register of British Acupuncturists (see 'Resources') will also satisfy the first and second points, as will nurse acupunc-turists, and they are also able to contact a patients's GP should this be necessary. Such acupuncturists will have trained for at least two years (full-time or part-time equivalent).

Patients must decide for themselves from whom they would prefer to receive acupuncture treatment, and nurses must decide whether they would satisfy their *Code of Professional Conduct* if they treated patients with such a complex and potentially dangerous form of medicine as acupuncture after only a few weekends of practical instruction.

In 1993 the National Association of Health Authorities and Trusts published the results of a national survey of purchasers (NAHAT 1993), which examined their attitudes towards the availability of complementary therapies in the NHS. More than 70 per cent of family health services authorities (FHSAs) and GP fundholders (GPFHs) and 65 per cent of district health authorities (DHAs) were in favour of some or all complementary therapies being available on the NHS, and thus free at the point of contact. Of those purchasers who were in favour, more than 90 per cent of FHSAs thought acupuncture should be available on the NHS, as did 80 per cent of GPFHs and 60 per cent of DHAs. Some 63 health-promotion clinics offering acupuncture had been approved by FHSAs; these clinics were mostly using acupuncture for help in giving up smoking and for pain relief. Other areas where acupuncture is being used in the NHS include radiotherapy, oncology, care of the elderly, psychiatry, anaesthetics, and physiotherapy.

The NAHAT survey found that 26 DHAs had contracts for acupuncture which were part of mainstream specialty contracts, and 2 had separate contracts. Of the GPFH practices, 23 offered acupuncture. The majority of therapies were provided by a member of the primary health-care team.

Examples of the use of acupuncture in nursing and health care

In midwifery

The Midwifery Acupuncture Unit at Freedom Fields Hospital in Plymouth was set up in 1988 and is under so much pressure that it cannot accept any new patients. Sarah Budd, a midwife and qualified acupuncturist working at the hospital, has used moxibustion with about two hundred women whose baby is in a breech presentation. She has achieved 60–5 per cent success in turning babies at 36–7 weeks. In China rates of 85–90 per cent have been recorded.

The hospital has now set up a trial to investigate the use of moxibustion in turning breech babies. In the first stage videos of ultrasound scans taken during moxibustion will be analysed by specialists in foetal behaviour to examine how it might be affecting the baby's movements. The second phase will be a large-scale trial, comparing the number of breech babies who turn after moxibustion at 34 weeks with the number who turn spontaneously. The maternity unit also offers acupuncture for pain relief during labour, and Ms Budd has visited China to investigate the use of acupuncture in Caesarean sections.

– Fursland, E. 1992. How to do a baby a good turn. *The Independent*,
August 11.

In physiotherapy

Nearly five hundred physiotherapists are known to be using
acupuncture in their practice both in the NHS and in the private
sector, primarily as a means of relieving pain.

– Hopwood, V. 1993. Acupuncture in physiotherapy. *Complementary
Therapies in Medicine* (April), 1(2): 100–3.

In giving up smoking

The method usually used in smoking clinics involves needles being
inserted in the ear at different points and then taped over. When
the patient wants a cigarette he or she taps the needles: this sends
a message to the addictive centre of the brain, which in turn stops
the craving for a cigarette. Success rates of 70 per cent have been
claimed by various clinics.

In pain clinics

Many pain clinics now offer acupuncture to patients. For example,
17 consecutive chronic back-pain patients attending Charing Cross
Hospital's Pain Relief Clinic in London were divided into two
groups: acupuncture and placebo. Both groups were examined for
tender points in such structures as the interspinous ligaments and
muscles of the spine and lower limbs. In the acupuncture group,
needles were inserted subcutaneously and painlessly into areas
overlying tender regions. The placebo group had inert electrodes
attached to an 'impressive-looking' piece of electrical apparatus,
but no electricity passed down the wires.

According to the researchers, 'the trial was of necessity single-
blind; nevertheless, it showed unequivocally that acupuncture
carried out in this way can have a beneficial effect'. Of back-pain
sufferers at the clinic, 47 per cent had relief for two months or
more following acupuncture.

– Macdonald, A. 1986. Getting under the skin. *Nursing Times* (May 14),
82: 47–8.

In child health

The Foundation of Traditional Medicine in Brighton holds a children's clinic which treats children with acupuncture, supplemented by herbal remedies. The most common ailments treated
are asthma, night screaming, colic and eczema.

– Caborn, A. 1988. Point taken. *Nursing Times* **84**(10): 31–3.

In the treatment of AIDS

The Acupuncture Clinic at the Lincoln Hospital in the Bronx, New York, has been using acupuncture in the treatment of AIDS since 1982. Patients with AIDS-related complex (ARC) have reported the following positive effects of acupuncture: increased energy, greater calmness, decreased size of nodes, increased sense of well-being, improved respiratory status, decreased night sweats, decreased diarrhoea, deceased size of a presumed lymphatic mass, and discontinued drug or alcohol abuse. Similar benefits were reported by patients with AIDS, who additionally reported increases in appetite and weight gain, and less toxicity from chemotherapy.

In the primary health-care setting

An acupuncture and osteopathy service has been offered free of charge to patients at the Wells Park general practice in Sydenham, South London. The acupuncturist and the osteopath work for one day each week of seven and six hours respectively, in one of the practice's treatment rooms. Between May 1987 and August 1988 the acupuncturist saw 90 patients and the osteopath 107.

– Budd, C., B. Fisher, D. Parrinder & L. Price 1990. A model of cooperation between complementary and allopathic medicine in a primary care setting. *British Journal of General Practice* **40**: 376–8.

Resources

Training and regulation

As the law stands at the moment, anyone can practise acupuncture regardless of whether or not they are qualified. However, it is possible to check whether an acupuncturist has appropriate qualifications. In 1982 the Register of British Acupuncturists was set up, combining the registers of the main professional organisations for qualified lay practitioners in the UK: the British Acupuncture Association, the International Register of Oriental Medicine (UK), the Register of Traditional Chinese Medicine, the Traditional Acupuncture Society, and the Chung San Acupuncture Society. Copies of the combined register are available from:

The Council for Acupuncture (CFA)
179 Gloucester Place, London NW1 6DZ.

Send a cheque for £2.00 and a large SAE.

Although each organisation has its own identity, all are bound by a common code of ethics and are covered by a block professional and public liability insurance policy. They also meet regularly as the Council for Acupuncture (CFA), which represents the profession as a whole both at national and local levels. The Council for Acupuncture was officially elected as the representative of the acupuncture profession in the UK in 1993; all queries relating to acupuncture can now be directed to one body. Member associations follow the CFA's directives on correct procedures for effective sterilisation of acupuncture equipment and needles, approved by the government. The CFA's aims are:

- to maintain high standards of education and training;
- to organise research;
- to promote acupuncture;
- to safeguard the public;
- to formulate codes of ethics and practice;
- to create links with the Department of Health, the BMA and the NHS.

The Council is also a member of the umbrella organisation, the Council for Complementary and Alternative Medicine (see Chapter 1), and of the World Federation of Acupuncture Societies.

In 1989 the Council for Acupuncture set up the British Acupuncture Accreditation Board (BAAB), which has developed a rigorous programme for acupuncture education which member organisations and their associated schools should meet (Shifrin 1993). All courses are at least two years (full-time or part-time equivalent) in length. BAAB assesses compliance with established minimum standards in colleges and the courses in acupuncture they run.

Useful addresses

British Acupuncture Association and Register (BAAR)
34 Alderney Street, London SW1V 4EU.

Chung San Acupuncture Society (CSAS)
15 Porchester Gardens, London W2 4DB.

International Register of Oriental Medicine (UK) (IROM)
Green Hedges House, Green Hedges Avenue, East Grinstead, West Sussex RH19 1DZ.

Register of Traditional Chinese Medicine (RTCM)
19 Trinity Road, London N2 8JJ.

Traditional Acupuncture Society (TAS)
1 The Ridgeway, Stratford-upon-Avon, Warwickshire CV37 9JL.

Medically qualified doctors have also begun to practise acupuncture, and in 1980 formed the British Medical Acupuncture Society. For more information, write to:

British Medical Acupuncture Society (BMAS)
Newton House, Newton Lane, Whitley, Warrington, Cheshire WA4 4JA.

Other acupuncture organisations include:

Association of Irish Acupuncturists (AIA)
PO Box 124, Tralee, Co. Kerry, Eire.

Association of Western Acupuncture (AWA)
12 Rodney Street, Liverpool LT2 2TE.

Electroacupuncture according to the Voll Society of Britain and Ireland
'Newnham', 15 Nower Hill, Pinner, Middlesex HA5 5QR.

(Members are mainly doctors.)

Recommended reading

- Beau, G. 1972. *Chinese Medicine*. New York: Avon Books.
- Kaptchuk, T. J. 1983. *The Web that has no Weaver*. London: Rider.
- Lawson-Wood, D. & J. Lawson-Wood 1974. *The Incredible Healing Needles*. New York: Samuel Weisner.
- Leger, J.-P. 1982. *The Little Red Book of Acupuncture*. Wellingborough: Thorsons.
- Lewith, G. T. 1982. *Acupuncture: its place in Western medical science*. Wellingborough: Thorsons.
- Macdonald, A. 1984. *Acupuncture: from ancient art to modern medicine*. London: Unwin.
- Maciocia, G. 1989. *The Foundation of Chinese Medicine: a comprehensive text for acupuncturists and herbalists*. Edinburgh: Churchill Livingstone.
- Mann, F. B. 1980. *Acupuncture: the ancient Chinese art of healing*. London: William Heinemann Medical.
- Mao-liang, Q. 1993. *Chinese Acupuncture and Moxibustion*. Edinburgh: Churchill Livingstone.
- Marcus, P. 1984. *Acupuncture: a patient's guide*. Wellingborough: Thorsons.
- Mole, P. 1992. *Acupuncture: energy balancing for body, mind and spirit*. Shaftesbury: Element.

- O'Connor, J. & D. Bensky (trans. and eds) 1984. *Acupuncture: a comprehensive text*. Shanghai: Shanghai College of Traditional Medicine (Seattle: Eastman Press).
- Wiseman, N., A. Ellis & P. Zmiewski 1985. *Fundamentals of Chinese Medicine*. Brookline, Massachusetts: Paradigm.
- Worsley, J. R. 1974. *Everyone's Guide to Acupuncture*. London: Cassell.
- Xinnong, C. (ed.) 1987. *Chinese Acupuncture and Moxibustion*. Beijing: Foreign Languages Press.

Chinese herbs

The use of herbs in Chinese medicine has a long history, and more has been written on the subject than about acupuncture.

Chinese herbalism, like acupuncture, involves a system based on the Taoist principles of Yin/Yang, balance, and the flow of nature. The emphasis in the use of herbs is on creating and maintaining health – **the Art of Radiant Health**, as the Chinese call it.

Through thousands of years of observation and study, the Chinese have classified hundreds of herbs. These herbs are divided into two categories:

- those which are 'building' – that is, those which help improve specific types of energy (for example, ginseng increases Qi);
- those which are 'clearing' (for example, herbs which clear heat in febrile conditions).

Building, or 'tonic', herbs can be taken as supplements to maintain good health. They are generally thought to taste good and are easily consumable. The qualities of tonic herbs include:

- increasing longevity by increasing well-being, strength and clarity of mind;
- enhancing psychological well-being;
- having no side-effects when used prudently, thereby abiding by the first rule of Chinese medicine – 'do no harm'.

Tonic herbs are believed by the Chinese to be important in building up the immune system. Over sixty tonic herbs have been identified as immune-system potentiators, including Astragalus, which has been investigated by the American Cancer Society. The main Chinese tonic herbs include:

- Wild Chinese Ginseng: Shen and Qi tonic;
- Chinese Ginseng: Qi tonic;
- Astragalus: Qi tonic;
- Ganoderma: Shen tonic;
- Schizandra: Yin tonic;

- Lycium: Yin tonic;
- Spirit Poria: Shen tonic and Qi tonic;
- Tang Kwei: Blood tonic;
- Deer Antler: Jing, Qi and Shen tonic.

Clearing herbs should only be taken under careful supervision over a short, prescribed period.

The art of professional Chinese herbalist is in the combining of herbs. Each prescription is based on a sophisticated diagnosis, and is individually tailored to each patient's needs. Herbs are used in prescriptions in such a way that the properties of the herbs that are needed to treat the condition are enhanced, and those properties of the herbs that may be unhelpful for the particular problem being treated are eliminated. A Chinese herbalist will also try to treat more than one aspect of the patient's problem with the herbal prescription. The prescription may thus include both clearing and building herbs.

As with acupuncture, the Chinese herbalist is always considering the symptoms and deep causes of the systems alongside each other, and treatment always seeks to tackle the cause of the problem.

In the UK, Chinese herbs are probably best known for their success in treating eczema, after the publicity surrounding Dr Ding Ho Luo, a Chinese herbalist who has been treating eczema, with a 75–85 per cent success rate, from her Soho surgery in London, since 1981 (Sadler 1992).

When her success came to the attention of David Atherton, consultant in paediatric dermatology at the Hospital for Sick Children, Great Ormond Street, London, he teamed up with a another consultant dermatologist at the hospital, Mary Sheehan, and undertook a placebo-controlled, double-blind trial with 47 children they were treating for severe, widespread, non-exudative atopic eczema. A limited number of standardised herbal formulae devised by Dr Luo were prescribed for these children rather than the conventional treatment options.

The results suggested that the active herbal treatment was much more effective than the placebo, with most children's eczema showing a 60 per cent improvement within four weeks of starting the active treatment. The children also suffered no side-effects (Atherton & Sheehan 1992; Sheehan 1992). A further trial at the Royal Free Hospital, London, has supported these findings. Dr Atherton is now involved in a trial which will offer liver tests to all patients attending the Chi Centre, a private clinic in Putney, to see whether any side-effects result from the use of Chinese herbs.

Interestingly, the eczema of some children did not benefit from the standardised formulae, but when an *individualised* prescription was given – perhaps with only one additional herb included – the

problem cleared up. This demonstrates the importance of individualised diagnosis and prescription, and highlights the way in which
in the West we persist in trying to standardise treatments rather
than to personalise them, despite our recognition that we are all
different.

Further reading

- Hsu, H. & W. G. Peacher 1976. *Chinese Herb Medicine and Therapy.* Los
  Angeles: Oriental Healing Arts.
- Toguchi, M. 1977. *Oriental Herbal Wisdom: a modern guide to the history,
  traditions, treatment and present practice of the world's most ancient form of
  healing.* New York: Pyramid Publications.

Resources

Chinese herbs

Register of Chinese Herbal Medicine (RCHM)
21 Warbeck Road, London W12 8NS.

The Register was formed in 1987 and is the professional body
representing practitioners practising Chinese herbal medicine in
the UK. All members are also qualified acupuncturists, and must
abide by the standards set by the Register. The Register also offers
insurance for members.

References

- Atherton, D. J., & M. P. Sheehan 1992. A controlled trial of traditional
  Chinese medicinal plants in widespread non-exudative atopic eczema.
  British Journal of Dermatology **126**: 179–84.
- Becker, R. O. 1974. The significance of bio-electric potentials.
  Bioelectrochemical Bioenergetics **1**: 187–99.
- Churchill, W. 1988. The point of health. *Nursing Times* **84**(44): 38–9.
- Darras, J., P. de Vernejoul & P. Albarede 1992. Nuclear medicine and
  acupuncture: a study on the migration of radioactive tracers after injec-
  tion at acupoints. *American Journal of Acupuncture* **20**(3): 245–55.
- Jessel-Kenyon, J., Ni Cheng, B. Blott & V. Hopwood 1992. Studies with
  acupuncture using a SQUID bio-magnetometer: a preliminary report.
  Complementary Medical Research **6**(3): 142–51.
- Lu, G., J. Xie, Y. Yang, *et al.* 1981. Afferent nerve fibre composition at
  point Zusanli in relation to acupuncture analgesia. *Chinese Medical
  Journal* **94**(4): 255–63.

– Mayer, D. J., D. D. Price & A. Rafii 1977. Antagonism of acupuncture analgesia in man by the narcotic naloxone. *Brain Research* **121**: 368–72.
– Melzack, R. 1978. Pain mechanisms: recent research. *Acupuncture Electro-therapy Research Journal* **3**: 109–12.
– Mole, P. 1992. *Acupuncture: energy balancing for the body, mind and spirit.* Shaftesbury: Element.
– NAHAT 1993. *Complementary Therapies in the NHS* (Research Paper No. 10). London: National Association of Health Authorities and Trusts.
– Price, P. & H. Rees 1982. The chemical basis of acupuncture analgesia. *British Journal of Acupuncture* **5**(2). 13–15.
– Sadler, C. 1992. Time for tea? *Nursing Times* **88**(35): 34–6.
– Sheehan, M. P. *et al.* 1992. Efficacy of traditional Chinese herbal therapy in adult atopic dermatitis. *Lancet* **340**: 13–17.
– Shifrin, K. 1993. Setting standards for acupuncture training – a model for complementary medicine. *Complementary Therapies in Medicine* **1**(2): 91–2.
– Zhang, A., X. Pan, J. Cheng, & W. Mo 1980. Endorphins and acupuncture analgesia. *Chinese Medical Journal* **93**(10): 673–80.

14 CHIROPRACTIC

Historical background

Spinal manipulation as a therapy has existed since at least Hippocrates' time, and possibly much earlier; variations, such as the native American practice of 'backwalking', have been noted in many cultures. In Europe during the Middle Ages there arose a group of healers known as 'bonesetters', who practised manipulation of joints for a range of ailments, and they flourished in Britain until the early years of the 20th century. In the last quarter of the 19th century, in the USA, a form of spinal manipulation called 'osteopathy' (see Chapter 15) appeared, which was to win many adherents.

Chiropractic (from the Greek *cheiro* and *praktikos*, meaning 'done by hand') was the invention of a Canadian, Daniel David Palmer. Between 1886 and 1895 he practised as a 'magnetic healer' in Iowa, but he had a special interest in the spine, and developed a theory that misalignments of the vertebrae could be at the root of many medical conditions.

In 1895 – 21 years after osteopathy was first developed – Palmer performed his first known chiropractic treatment. A man who said he had been deaf for 17 years following an incident when he hurt his neck in lifting, received three manipulations, and – the story goes – hearing was returned.

Palmer set up a school ('Dr Palmer's School and Cure', later 'The Palmer Institute and Chiropractic Infirmary) in Davenport, Iowa, and was imprisoned for practising medicine without a licence. His son, Bartlett Joshua Palmer, developed the theory further, but several schisms among groups of practitioners occurred in the early 1920s and beyond.

The first US State licence was granted by Kansas in 1913; now all US states recognise chiropractic as a valid therapy, as do Australia, New Zealand, and several other countries. In Europe, only Switzerland, Norway and Liechtenstein (and, until its split, the former Yugoslavia) have chiropractic legislation.

The growth of chiropractic's acceptance in the USA is an interesting story. In 1963, the American Medical Association (AMA) formed a 'Committee on Quackery', and their final verdict on chiropractic was that it was 'an unscientific cult'. As one author noted,'... the hostility of the medical establishment forced chiropractic to get its scientific act together' (Olsen 1991), so well, in fact, that in 1974 chiropractic treatment was admitted to the list of therapies covered by Medicaid, the safety-net medical insurance scheme; and (also in 1974) the US Commission on Education gave the American Chiropractic Association the right to accredit training courses, which could then apply for federal funding. The AMA withdrew their use of the word 'unscientific' in relation to chiropractic, and in 1987 the American Hospitals Association allowed licensed chiropractors to use hospital facilities.

The British Chiropractors' Association, forerunner of the British Chiropractic Association (BCA), was formed in 1925, and the therapy enjoyed some success until the founding of the National Health Service in 1948 saw the end of the Approved Health Insurance Societies, many of which had been willing to pay for chiropractic treatment. Under the new rules, only treatment provided within the NHS was free to users. An application by the BCA to join the NHS in 1974 was rejected, but the profession received a boost three years later when the General Medical Council ruled that, providing doctors retained ultimate clinical responsibility, they could officially refer their patients to a chiropractor when appropriate.

A major survey of the use of 'non-orthodox' therapies, undertaken by public-health researchers at Sheffield University and published in the *British Medical Journal* in 1991 (Thomas *et al.* 1991), found that over three-quarters of people seeking help from complementary therapists did so for musculoskeletal problems; this suggests that there is considerable demand for the kind of therapy that chiropractors offer.

In the UK, anyone can call him- or herself a chiropractor, but there are registers of qualified practitioners (see 'Resources') which can be consulted, and it seems likely that statutory regulation will be enforced in the near future.

Further reading

- Copland-Griffiths, M. 1991. *Dynamic Chiropractic Today*. Wellingborough: Thorsons.
- Inglis, B. 1979. *Natural Medicine*. London: Collins.
- Mills, S. 1993. The development of the complementary medical professions. *Complementary Therapies in Medicine* 1(1): 24–9.
- Moore, S. 1988. *Chiropractic*. London: Macdonald Optima.

What is chiropractic?

In May 1993, the Kings Fund called for legislation that would put chiropractors on a par with nurses, midwives and health visitors in terms of professional regulation and protection of their title. Even the British Medical Association (1993), not previously noted for a sympathetic stance regarding complementary therapies, included chiropractic in its list of discrete clinical disciplines, '... the therapies which have established foundations of training and have the potential for greatest use alongside orthodox medical care'. In February 1994 the possibility of a chiropractors bill was discussed in the House of Commons.

How it works

The theory behind **chiropractic** is, on the surface, quite simple: if there is any misalignment of the vertebrae, leading to restricted, excessive, or in any way abnormal movement within the spinal column (Figure 14.1), then the result will be a bodily malfunction. The spine, chiropractors point out, provides protection for a large part of the central nervous system – the spinal cord – and although the link is not always completely understood, problems with vertebral alignment can manifest themselves in a whole range of sensory, organic, vascular and muscular problems. Chiropractic involves manipulation of joints, with the aim of restoring alignment, and a teacher of the technique suggests that this works on three levels:

- *Mechanical/anatomical* Restoring movement by improving anatomical relationships and functions through a variety of spinal-manipulation and joint-mobilisation techniques.
- *Neurological/reflexive* Specific soft- and hard-tissue (joint muscles and fascia) manipulations can change nerve signalling patterns and, therefore, physiological functioning.
- *Mental/emotional role* The healing aspects of human contact, its hands-on methodology, and its effects on the mind and motivation of a patient, are part of the overall benefits.

Joints other than the spine may be treated, as will be seen below.

Chiropractors use the term **biomechanics** in explaining their techniques; this implies that mechanical function (or dysfunction) in the body is intimately related to biological function, both in health and illness.

The aim of treatment is to identify any areas of the spine where movement is in any way abnormal; to establish the reason or reasons for this abnormality; and, if manipulation is an appropriate treatment, to attempt to restore normal movement. Further discussion of this concept can be found under 'Visiting a chiropractor'.

As with naturopathy (see Chapter 12), chiropractic aims to supplement the body's own defences by restoring the homoeostatic balance, which the earliest chiropractors called **innate intelligence**.

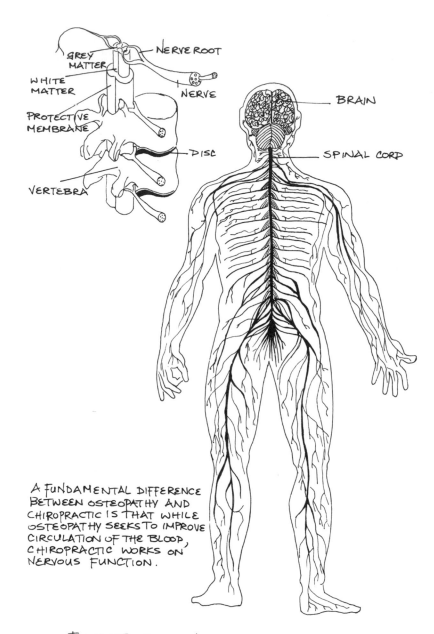

GREY MATTER

WHITE MATTER

PROTECTIVE MEMBRANE

VERTEBRA

NERVE ROOT

NERVE

DISC

BRAIN

SPINAL CORD

A FUNDAMENTAL DIFFERENCE BETWEEN OSTEOPATHY AND CHIROPRACTIC IS THAT WHILE OSTEOPATHY SEEKS TO IMPROVE CIRCULATION OF THE BLOOD, CHIROPRACTIC WORKS ON NERVOUS FUNCTION.

FIG 14.1: THE CENTRAL NERVOUS SYSTEM AND THE SPINE

Visiting a chiropractor

The first two steps in treatment are the collection of a detailed history, including as much information as possible about the person's lifestyle, and a series of general observations of posture and gait. After this, the principal diagnostic tools used are, unsurprisingly, the practitioner's hands, but X-rays also are widely used. Chiropractors are extremely cautious about inappropriate treatment, and may well, at this stage, refer the patient to a doctor if the condition is not one amenable to chiropractic (see 'Contra-indications').

Once a diagnosis has been reached, a treatment régime can begin. This may include:

- **Mobilisation** The person is asked to move the joint as far as possible, until he or she reaches the end of the range of active movement. Mobilisation involves the chiropractor exerting enough force to take the joint a little further, until the end of the range of passive movement is reached.
- **Manipulation** When a joint has been passively moved as far as it will go, the resistance encountered can be overcome by manipulation, in which further force is applied until the joint surfaces are moved apart. This may be accompanied by a 'cracking' noise, like that made by people 'cracking their knuckles', as carbon dioxide is freed from the synovial fluid which bathes the joint.

Manipulation – or **adjustment**, as it is sometimes called – is a precise skill: a very slight over-exertion of force could damage the joint.

There are thirty-six different adjustments (Copland-Griffiths 1991), but the two most used are classed as *dynamic* (high-velocity thrust) or *recoil*. A chiropractor describes the difference like this (Moore 1988, pp. 61–2):

> In a recoil adjustment, the patient usually lies in a neutral and relaxed position, often face down on the treatment table. The chiropractor makes contact with the edge of her palm on a specific joint to be adjusted and removes any slack from the skin so a tight contact is obtained. She gives a very fast thrust to the joint through the contact of her hand on the surface of the skin. This thrust has a high speed, but a low amplitude or depth in order to avoid any damage to the structures in the area.
>
> With the dynamic or high-velocity thrust adjustment, the part of the body being adjusted has to be positioned so that the joint is at the limit of its active range of motion. For the low back, this requires the patient to lie on one side with the upper body twisted in the opposite direction to the pelvis, to introduce an element of rotation and lateral flexion to the spine. This in turn brings the spinal joints to the limit of their active range of movement. By causing a counter-rotation on the spine,

achieved by varying the extent to which the hips and knees are bent, a point of tension can be obtained at which the chiropractor makes a specific contact with her hand on the area to be adjusted. She then carefully turns the patient's body so that the joint is taken through its range of movement to the elastic barrier of resistance [the point at which manipulation needs to be applied, if further movement is to be effected]. The chiropractor applies a small thrust, again of high speed but short amplitude. The thrust is given in a specific direction in order to restore normal spinal and joint mechanics, function and integrity. It may be necessary to repeat this action at more than one level in the lumbar spine and first on one side and then the other.

What the chiropractor is treating is a perceived alteration in the normal function of a joint or joints; this is sometimes called a **fixation**. This does not mean that the joint is actually 'fixed', or immobile; rather, that there is some degree of restriction on normal movement, which in turn can have effects on tissues at some distance from it. Fixations can be divided into three types:

- **Static motor unit fixations** The joint is fixed in flexion, extension, lateral flexion, or rotation.
- **Kinetic motor unit fixations** The joint cannot move freely – it is *hypomobile* – and to compensate, other motor units become *hypermobile*.
- **Structural alterations** As the term implies, the fixation results from an alteration in the spine's normal shape (for example, kyphosis, or 'dowager's hump', in which the thoracic spine curves outwards, or scoliosis, in which the spine curves sideways). Postural problems may also be implicated.

Chiropractors believe that the causes of fixations fall into three groups:

- *mechanical* – examples of this are trauma, and the use of badly-designed chairs and beds;
- *chemical* – this includes allergic reactions and nutritional problems;
- *psychological* – the chief of these is stress.

Establishing the cause of the presenting problem is a priority in the chiropractor's initial assessment; with this grouping of causes, it can be seen that the history-taking has to be very wide-ranging, to elicit all relevant information.

Indications

About 50 per cent of all chiropractic consultations are made because of low back pain, including hip problems; and around

40 per cent deal with head, neck and chest pain, including cervical spondylosis and migraines. The remainder comprises people seeking treatment for wrist, ankle, knee and elbow problems, and for health problems that do not, at first sight, appear to have much connection with joints, such as asthma, dysmenorrhoea, and disorders of the gastro-intestinal tract (Moore 1988; Copland-Griffiths 1991); chiropractors believe that such conditions can result from fixations.

Contra-indications

Because of the damage that can be caused by spinal manipulation, qualified practitioners are very careful about what conditions they treat.

Inflammation in, and infections of, the spine, and any neoplastic disease in the area, are absolute contra-indications (Copland-Griffiths 1991). Osteoporosis, ligament damage, and fractures call for the avoidance of certain techniques; and circulatory problems such as the presence of an aneurysm, or advanced arteriosclerotic disease, also impose a requirement for extra caution in treatment.

Research

B. J. Palmer established a research centre in 1935 in the USA, and although his work lacked the hallmarks of scientific rigour expected today, 'the seeds of research planted by him ... were reaped in the 1970s and 1980s when a small band of researchers applied scientific principles to the examination of chiropractic theories, this time to dramatic and positive effect' (Copland-Griffiths 1991). The Canadian Memorial Chiropractic College in Toronto established the Chiropractic Research Abstracts Collection (CRAC), which forms an index of international research, in 1974; a 1985 publication listed 120 books available in English (West & Trevelyan 1985); and in 1986 *The Chiropractic Theories – a synopsis of scientific research* was published (Leach 1986).

Chiropractors acknowledge the need for properly conducted clinical evaluation of their therapy (Moore 1988), and all students undertaking the BCA recognised training at the Anglo-European College of Chiropractic (see 'Resources') undertake research as a course requirement.

A frequently-cited piece of recent research is discussed in Box 14.1.

BOX 14.1
CHIROPRACTIC AND LOWER BACK PAIN

Perhaps the most complete recent research project carried out in Britain was one carried out by Medical Research Council epidemiologists and a rheumatologist, whose results were published in the *British Medical Journal* in 1990.

In a randomised, controlled, multi-centre trial, 741 patients, aged between 18 and 65, all having severe lower back pain of mechanical origin, received either chiropractic (from BCA registered practitioners) or hospital out-patient treatment. The chiropractors were to give no more than ten treatments, preferably within a three-month period but spread over a year if necessary; the paper does not give details of any constraints on the hospital teams.

Progress was measured using the results of the Oswestry pain disability questionnaire (a recognised and validated research tool), and tests of straight leg raising and lumbar flexion exercises. Follow-up was initially planned to last for two years.

The results showed that with the Oswestry scores, only one hospital department (out of eleven) appeared to get better results than chiropractors, and results were equivocal in two more, leaving eight centres at which chiropractic was significantly more effective. With leg raising and lumbar flexion, patients treated by chiropractors did better than those treated as hospital out-patients.

The comparative benefits of chiropractic became more marked at six months into the follow-up period, and as a result the researchers extended this by another year. The improvements – including a decreased chance of needing further treatment – were maintained. The authors concluded:

> For patients with low back pain in whom manipulation is not contra-indicated, chiropractic almost certainly confers worthwhile, long-term benefit in comparison with hospital out-patient management. The benefit is mainly seen in those with chronic or severe pain. Introducing chiropractic into NHS practice should be considered.

– Meade, T. W., S. Dyer, W. Browne, *et al.* 1990. Low back pain of mechanical origin: randomised comparison of chiropractic and hospital outpatient treatment. *British Medical Journal* 300(6770): 1431–7.

The principal author published another paper, summarising the findings of this study and proposing the additional idea that physiotherapists be trained in chiropractic technique.

– Meade, T. W. 1990. Chiropractic treatment of low back pain. *MRC News* (September), 48: 23–4.

CHIROPRACTIC AND OSTEOPATHY

It is difficult for the non-specialist to see the differences between chiropractic and osteopathy at first, but they do exist. D. D. Palmer wrote: 'Chiropractic resembles osteopathy more so than any other method, yet they are as different as day is from night ... [their respective philosophies] are radically and entirely different'. The most fundamental difference is that osteopathy's benefits are said to be due to improved circulation of the blood, while in chiropractic it is nervous function that is thought to be affected (Copland-Griffiths 1991).

Techniques differ, too. One chiropractor describes it thus (Howitt Wilson 1991):

The chiropractor uses rapid, low-amplitude thrusts directly onto one of the bones adjacent to a joint. The point of contact is on the vertebra to be moved, and speed is of the essence. He may use other techniques, but his adjustments are such that they can be performed with little or no preparation. The osteopath does more soft-tissue work (superficial and deep massage), mobilises the joints by traction or articulation (putting joints through their full range of movement passively) and finally may deliver a more specific thrust, after a long-lever move with the point of contact at a distance from the joint to be moved.

Implications for nursing

Chiropractic is a highly-skilled therapy, requiring the equivalent of six years' full-time study in the largest training establishment, and continuous clinical practice; other branches of the discipline, where the training is shorter, are likely to move towards this extended course in the near future. There are *no* chiropractic techniques which an untrained person could safely perform on another; but nurses need to know something about the therapy because as its profile rises in coming years, following osteopathy away from the fringes of medical practice and into the 'orthodox' arena, patients and clients may well turn to them for information.

Training and regulation

Currently, anybody can call themselves a chiropractor in this country. To confuse matters still further, there is more than one form of training.

Until statutory regulation is introduced, however – and after the Kings Fund report of May 1993, backing the profession's call for such regulation, and the passing of the Osteopaths Act in July of the same year, it seems likely that it will be – there is one British college whose course is recognised by the British Chiropractic Association (BCA), the European Chiropractors' Union, and affiliated international organisations: the Anglo-European College of Chiropractic (details below). This leads to the award of Doctor of Chiropractic (DC). Five years' training, which has been accorded BSc status by the Council for National Academic Awards, is followed by a mandatory postgraduate year, similar to that which doctors of medicine undertake.

The BCA has a code of practice to which members must adhere, and its disciplinary committee has the power to reprimand, fine, or remove from its register, any member against whom a complaint is upheld.

Details of BCA registered chiropractors can be obtained from:

British Chiropractic Association (BCA)
29 Whitley Street, Reading, Berkshire RG2 0EG.

European Chiropractors Union (ECU)
82 Waldegrave Road, Teddington, Middlesex TW11 8LG.

Details of chiropractic training can be obtained from:

Anglo-European College of Chiropractic (AECC)
13–15 Parkwood Road, Bournemouth BH5 2DF.

There is a particular form of chiropractic known as **McTimoney**, recognised by a body called The Institute of Pure Chiropractic. The main difference between McTimoney and chiropractic as taught as the Anglo-European college is that the technique is based on a manoeuvre called the **toggle recoil**, D. D. Palmer's 'original technique that was lost'. Interestingly, the technique is also used in veterinary practice.

Practitioners qualified in this form of chiropractic use the initials MC (McTimoney Chiropractor) or AMC (Animal McTimoney

Chiropractor) after their names. For three years after qualifying they can be associate members of the Institute, and use the letters AIPC, after which they may apply for full membership, becoming MIPC.

Details can be obtained from:

Institute of Pure Chiropractic (IPC)
14 Park End Street, Oxford OX1 1HH.

As the move towards statutory regulation gets nearer, it seems likely that chiropractors from the BCA, IPC, and a third group called **Witney chiropractors** will form closer links; but at the moment, no one can say what form any alliance might take.

Recommended reading

- Copland-Griffiths, M. 1991. *Dynamic Chiropractic Today*. Wellingborough: Thorsons.
- Howitt Wilson, M. B. 1991. *Chiropractic*, revd edn. London: Thorsons.
- Leach, R. A. 1986. *The Chiropractic Theories – a synopsis of scientific research*. Baltimore: Williams & Wilkins.
- Moore, S. 1988a. *A Guide to Chiropractic*. London: Hamlyn.
- Moore, S. 1988b. *Chiropractic*. London: Macdonald Optima.

References

- British Medical Association 1993. *Complementary Medicine: new approaches to good practice*. Oxford: Oxford University Press.
- Copland-Griffiths, M. 1991. *Dynamic Chiropractic Today*. Wellingborough: Thorsons.
- Howitt Wilson, M. B. 1991. *Chiropractic*, revd edn. London: Thorsons.
- Leach, R. A. 1986. *The Chiropractic Theories – a synopsis of scientific research*. Baltimore: Williams & Wilkins.
- Moore, S. 1988. *A Guide to Chiropractic*. London: Hamlyn.
- Olsen, K. 1991. *The Encyclopaedia of Alternative Medicine*. London: Piatkus.
- Thomas, K. J., J. Carr, L. Westlake, *et al.* 1991. Use of non-orthodox and conventional health care in Great Britain. *British Medical Journal* 302(6770): 207–10.
- West, R. & J. E. Trevelyan 1985. *Alternative Medicine – a bibliography of books in English*. London: Mansell.

15 OSTEOPATHY

Historical background

Osteopathy was developed in 1874 by an American, Andrew Taylor Still (1828–1912). Still worked as a doctor in a small town in the mid-West of America, where he had become increasingly disenchanted with medicine and its ability to help patients. He himself watched three of his own children die from cerebrospinal meningitis. The idea of osteopathy grew from Still's Christian faith, a sound practical knowledge of mechanics, and a history of inventing machinery. He saw the body as a machine made in God's likeness and therefore perfect in design. Such a machine, he argued, could only become ill if it got out of adjustment. Restoration of normal function could be made via the muscles and joints. Ailments which seemingly had nothing to do with the spine – such as headaches, skin disorders and digestive disorders – were, in Still's view, the result of the spinal column being out of position in some way. Therefore, he argued, manipulation of the spine that restored the proper alignment would successfully treat the condition.

Still began to write on the subject and to teach others of the methods of treatment he had developed. In 1892 he established the first teaching courses in osteopathy at Kirksville, Missouri. Soon after, he opened Kirksville College, which is still one of America's most important centres of osteopathic education and research.

One of Still's pupils was a Scot, James Martin Littlejohn, a graduate of Glasgow University with degrees in Law, Divinity and Arts. Littlejohn had moved to the USA in 1892 – the year Still opened his school – and received treatment from Still in 1897. In 1898 he enrolled as a student. Littlejohn went on to give the first ever lecture on osteopathy in England (for which he received the Gold Medal of the Society of Science, Letters and Arts). He became vice-principal at the Kirksville College, and in 1900 he established the American School of Osteopathic Medicine and Surgery in Chicago (now called the Chicago College of Osteopathic Medicine). Littlejohn returned to the UK in 1913 and in 1917 he set up the British School of Osteopathy. Some years later, other schools were also set up: the London College of Osteopathic Medicine in 1946, and the European School of Osteopathy in 1965.

Littlejohn had a holistic view of osteopathy and described it as the science of adjustment. He believed a person had to be in perfect balance not only with the physical world, but also with regard to diet and social, domestic and occupational factors. An osteopath's job, he argued, was to adjust the patient to normal in all these fields. This led to an expansion in the curriculum as well as in the concept of osteopathy.

From 1902, a small number of American osteopaths came to the UK to work. For the next twenty-five years there were more American osteopaths in the UK than British, and osteopaths struggled hard to gain recognition. Eventually in 1935 a Select Committee of the House of Lords found no reason to enact special legislation and advised the profession to put its own house in order. In 1936, therefore, the General Council and Register of Osteopaths was set up to monitor the education and practice of osteopaths.

During the 1930s an American osteopath, William Garner Sutherland, developed the technique of cranial osteopathy (see page 213).

Today, osteopathy is a well-known and well-established complementary therapy. Doctors refer patients to osteopaths, and many sporting teams and clubs use osteopaths as well as physiotherapists. There are now two schools offering a degree in osteopathy, and in 1995 osteopathy will become a regulated profession in the same way as those of nurses, doctors and dentists.

Further reading

- Chaitow, L. 1979. *Osteopathy: head-to-toe health through manipulation.* Wellingborough: Thorsons.
- Latey, P. 1993a. Osteopathy ancient and modern. *Journal of Osteopathic Education* (January), 3(1): 14–21.
- Latey, P. 1993b. Still and osteopathy before 1990. *Journal of Osteopathic Education* (January), 3(1): 9–12.
- Latey, P. 1993c. Thinking osteopathically in the early 1900s. *Journal of Osteopathic Education* (January), 3(1): 12–14.
- Still, A. T. 1897. *Autobiography of A. T. Still*, reprinted 1977. Colorado Springs, Colorado: American Academy of Osteopathy.

What is osteopathy?

Osteopathy, according to its founder, Andrew Taylor Still, 'is that science which consists of such exact exhaustive and verifiable knowledge of the structure and function of the human mechanism, anatomical, physiological and psychological, including chemistry and physics of its known elements, as has made discoverable certain organic laws and remedial resources, within the body itself, by which nature under the scientific treatment peculiar to osteopathic practice, apart from all ordinary methods of extraneous, artificial or medicinal stimulation, and in harmonious accord with its own mechanical principles, molecular activities and metabolic processes, may recover from displacements, disorganisations, derangements and consequent disease, and regain its normal equilibrium of form and function in health and strength' (Still 1897).

Putting it more simply, the Osteopathic Information Service (OIS – see 'Resources') describes osteopathy as 'a system of diagnosis and treatment which lays its main emphasis on the structural and mechanical problems of the body. It is not an alternative to conventional medicine but a complementary discipline which offers patients an additional treatment option for certain conditions which can affect the body's framework' (OIS: personal communication).

Still summarised the principles of osteopathy as 'structure governs function: that is, a problem in the mechanical structure of the body will impair its functioning (Figure 15.1). Still also believed that, given the right circumstances, the body has the power to heal itself.

The central elements of osteopathic philosophy can be summarised as follows:

- The body is a unit.
- Structure and function are reciprocally inter-related.
- The body possesses self-regulatory mechanisms.
- The body has the inherent capacity to defend itself and repair itself.
- When normal adaptability is disrupted, or when environmental changes overcome the body's capacity for self-maintenance, disease may ensue.
- Movement of body fluids is essential to the maintenance of health.
- The nerves play a crucial part in controlling the fluids of the body.
- There are somatic components to disease that are not only manifestations of disease but also factors that contribute to maintenance of the diseased state.

For a more detailed explanation of these concepts, see Giovanna and Schiowitz's book (1991).

Osteopaths, says Stephen Sandler (1992), 'are practitioners of manual medicine; in other words, they work with their hands both to diagnose conditions and to treat them. Osteopaths use palpation, feeling the tissues under their fingers, and by comparing the temperature, tone, shape and response to movement to what they know to be normal, decide how best to manually treat the patient'.

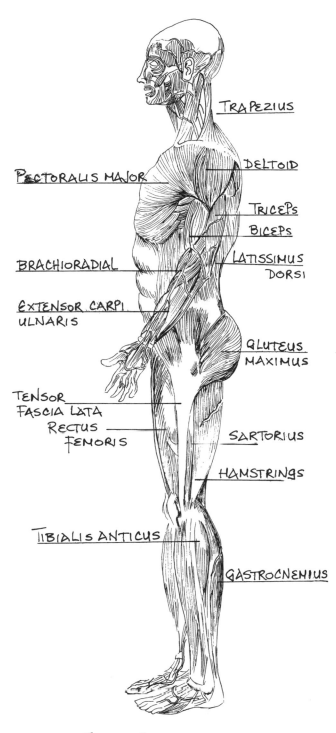

TRAPEZIUS

DELTOID

PECTORALIS MAJOR

TRICEPS

BICEPS

LATISSIMUS DORSI

BRACHIORADIAL

EXTENSOR CARPI ULNARIS

GLUTEUS MAXIMUS

TENSOR FASCIA LATA

RECTUS FEMORIS

SARTORIUS

HAMSTRINGS

TIBIALIS ANTICUS

GASTROCNEMIUS

Fig 15.1 : HUMAN MUSCULATURE

During the process of diagnosis, an osteopath will be trying to establish where the mechanical fault, or **osteopathic lesion**, lies. The word 'lesion' comes from the Latin *laedare*, which means 'to hurt'. In osteopathy, 'lesion' is used to describe a specific type of joint dysfunction, usually in the spinal column (Figure 15.2). An osteopathic lesion is a joint in which there is anything from slight to total limitation of normal physiological movement. Lesions may be caused by such things as injury, disease, or bad posture.

Every structure in the human body is connected either directly or indirectly to the spinal cord. However, osteopaths do not consider the spine to be the only factor in disease, and accept the importance of genetic, developmental, dietary, environmental, psychological and bacteriological factors. Osteopathy makes no claim to be able to treat conditions caused by these factors.

Types of treatment

There is a variety of different techniques which can be selected depending on the problem brought by the individual patient. Techniques are either 'direct' or 'indirect':

- **Direct techniques** include soft-tissue techniques, mobilisation techniques (passive and active), manipulation (low-amplitude and high-velocity thrust), muscle-energy technique, and myofascial technique.
- **Indirect techniques** include functional technique, strain–counterstrain technique, and cranio-sacral technique (involuntary mechanism).

For further information on these techniques, the following texts are helpful:

- Giovanna, E. L. & S. Schiowitz 1991. *An Osteopathic Approach to Diagnosis and Treatment*. Philadelphia, Pennsylvania: J. B. Lippincott.
- Hartman, L. 1983. *Handbook of Osteopathic Technique*. Hadley Wood, Hertfordshire: N. M. K. Publishers.
- Neumann, H. D. 1989. *Introduction to Manual Medicine*. Berlin: Springer Verlag.

Visiting an osteopath

At the first consultation, the osteopath will take a full case history, including the past medical history. A thorough physical examination follows, during which the osteopath will examine the patient's posture and the way he or she moves, observing any restriction or exaggeration in movement in any area. The patient's spine will be examined in detail, and the osteopath will test the movement of each vertebra, looking for tenderness, stiffness or

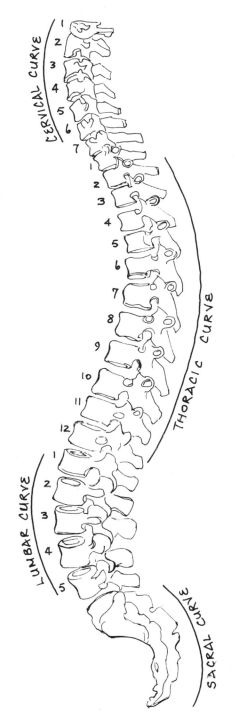

Fig 15.2 : THE SPINAL COLUMN

increased movement. Patients are asked to undress to their underwear for the physical examination and treatment, but the osteopath will be sensitive to any ethnic and religious restrictions. Osteopaths will refer a patient for conventional investigations such as X-rays or blood examinations if these are deemed necessary.

According to the College of Osteopathy (see 'Resources'):

> Patients who have not previously experienced osteopathic treatment are sometimes a little surprised and puzzled by the techniques of examination employed. Parts of the body apparently unrelated to the symptoms are often examined. For example, a patient may complain of pain down his arm and 'tingling' of the fingers, yet the osteopath focuses his attention on the lower part of the neck. This is because an osteopathic lesion in the cervical [neck] spine is often responsible for pressure on a nerve root causing pain to radiate down the arm.

This process of diagnosis will establish whether a patient can safely receive manipulation, which area of the body needs treatment, and what type of treatment should be given. An osteopath is well versed in orthopaedics and pathology and will recommend that a patient seeks help elsewhere if this would be more helpful.

Depending on which treatment programme the osteopath decides upon, the patient will be asked to lie on the treatment table in a position which will allow the osteopath to apply the right amount of force or leverage to get the tissue to change under his or her own hands. The treatment is not necessarily painful.

Osteopathic adjustments are often preceded by extensive soft-tissue work, which helps the muscles relax and permits easier movement of the joints. Indeed this may be all that is necessary. Joint adjustments are movements made passively through the normal physiological range of the particular joint. These movements may produce a characteristic 'click' but are not painful.

There may be some reaction one or two days after a treatment, which some patients describe as a 'bruised' feeling. This normally clears up by the third day.

How many treatments are necessary varies according to the patient. Some low-back conditions clear up after a only a couple of treatments, whereas other may take six or more. Some conditions are more or less permanent, but regular osteopathic treatment may bring relief and improved movement. Each session is usually around 20–30 minutes long, although the first appointment may be for an hour.

The osteopath may suggest alternative ways of going about daily tasks or exercises which may help with the problem being treated. Others, who may also have a qualification in naturopathy, may suggest dietary changes and other naturopathic therapies.

Indications

The two thousand osteopaths practising in the UK treat some 100 000 patients a week – half of them for back pain (Consumers Association 1993). Treatment is also given for tension headaches, neck and shoulder pain, and joint strain in shoulders, wrists, elbows, knees, ankles and feet.

The Osteopathic Information Service reports that 'many women also use osteopathic treatment as an alternative to drugs for the relief of aches, pain and discomfort often associated with pregnancy. Sports men and women will consult an osteopath following injuries, while others find treatment can alleviate problems which have previously prevented them from performing at their best'.

According to a *Which?* report (Consumers Association 1986), osteopathy has become the most widely used complementary therapy. The report also said that 82 per cent of patients using osteopathy said that their problem was cured or improved by the treatment.

Osteopaths also claim to be able to help with arthritis, asthma, sciatica, tenosynovitis (tennis elbow), tension headaches and migraines, frozen shoulder, cervical spondylosis, neuritis, rheumatic aches and pains, chronic respiratory ailments, and menstrual disorders.

Contra-indications

Osteopathic diagnosis and treatment is essentially manual, and there are no harmful side-effects. Osteopaths are taught to use minimal force to manipulate or move a patient's joint.

Osteopaths will recommend that pregnant women do not receive any osteopathic treatment during the period of pregnancy when the blood supply to the foetus changes from uterine to placental, as this is the period when spontaneous abortions are most likely. There is no evidence that osteopathy will cause a miscarriage, but osteopaths prefer to take this precautionary measure.

There are many physical conditions that osteopaths will treat with great caution, such as brittle bones and inflamed joints; and osteopaths do not claim to be able to cure conditions such as cancer or heart disease, although they will treat patients suffering from these conditions, to help them feel more relaxed and comfortable. Osteopaths are trained in differential diagnosis and will always tell a patient whether or not osteopathy is the most appropriate form of treatment, and when osteopathy cannot help.

Research

During the 1940s a physiologist called Professor Irvin Korr worked with osteopaths to investigate abnormal function in the spine. Using electrical measurements from within muscles, he recorded their increased activity and showed that some of the changes that osteopaths believe important (osteopathic lesions) were in fact real – something which, until then, many orthodox doctors had doubted (Campbell 1984).

Since then, a wide range of research projects has been undertaken to investigate the value and efficacy of osteopathy. A selection of published material is given below. Most colleges of osteopathy are committed to further research, and many students are actively involved in investigations as part of their courses.

- Burton, A. K., K. M. Tillotson, V. A. Edwards, *et al.* 1990. Lumbar sagittal mobility and low back symptoms in patients treated with manipulation. *Journal of Spinal Disorders* 3: 362–8.
- Cleary, C. 1990. Osteopathy and menopausal women. *Complementary Medical Research* 4(3): 60–1.
- Coleridge, S. T. 1991. Research and scholarly activities during osteopathic residency training. *Journal of the American Osteopathic Association* 91(9): 891–4.
- Ellestad, S. M., R. V. Nagle, D. R. Boesler, *et al.* 1988. Electromyographic and skin-resistance responses to osteopathic treatment for low back pain. *Journal of the American Osteopathic Association* 88(8): 991–7.
- Korr, I. M. 1991. Osteopathic research: the needed paradigm shift. *Journal of American Osteopathic Association* 91(2): 156–68.
- MacDonald, R. S. 1990. Open controlled assessment of osteopathic manipulation in non-specific low back pain. *Spine* 15(5): 364–70.
- Paul, F. A., J. M. Norton, N. A. Cross, *et al.* 1990. Effect of osteopathic treatment (OMT) on heart rate and blood pressure in female athletes. *Journal of Spinal Disorders* 3: 363–8.
- Szmelskyj, A. O. 1990. The difference between holistic osteopathic practice and manipulation. *Holistic Medicine* 5: 67–79.
- Szmelskyj, A. O. Qualifications and geographical distribution of practitioners of osteopathy. *Complementary Medical Research* 2(1): 10–18.
- Tyreman, S. 1992. Concepts for osteopathic health care (II). *Journal of Osteopathic Education* (January), 2(1): 10–18.

Implications for nursing

Osteopathy requires four years' full-time study and should not be practised in *any* form by untrained individuals. It is therefore unlikely to be widely incorporated within nursing practice. However, nurses should be aware of its value and can usefully suggest osteopathy to clients as a possible source of help. This advice should, however, be given only after discussion and agreement with the patient's doctor and after seeking general advice from a qualified osteopath.

In January 1975 the General Medical Council publicly stated that doctors could refer patients to osteopaths if they wished, providing they retained responsibility; and in 1978 a Dr Cyril Pragnell, a member of the then government's back-pain committee, went as far as to suggest that if hospitals were to establish osteopathic departments under the control of qualified osteopaths, the departments of orthopaedic medicine would soon disappear (Potterton 1978).

The Department of Health generally accepts sickness certificates from qualified osteopaths, as do most private health insurance companies (although osteopathy is covered by only a small number of insurance companies).

A study of Szmelskyj and Morris (1992) explored GPs' attitudes to, and knowledge of, osteopathy in the Huntingdon Health Authority area. Of the GPs who responded, 58 per cent claimed to understand the difference between osteopathy, physiotherapy and chiropractic. Most thought osteopathy useful in the treatment of mechanical and degenerative musculoskeletal problems, especially lumbar and spinal complaints.

In 1993 the National Association of Health Authorities and Trusts published the results of a national survey (NAHAT 1993) of district health authorities (DHAs), family health services authorities (FHSAs) and GP fundholders (GPFHs) to examine purchasers' attitudes towards the availability of complementary therapies in the NHS. More than 70 per cent of FHSAs and GPFHs, and 65 per cent of DHAs, were in favour of some or all complementary therapies being available on the NHS, and thus free at the point of contact. Of those purchasers who were in favour of making complementary therapies available on the NHS, 25 per cent of DHAs thought that osteopathy should be available, as did more than 75 per cent of FHSAs and GPFHs. Further, 21 health-promotion clinics using osteopathy have been approved by FHSAs.

Various co-operative links already exist between osteopaths and the health service. For example, students from the British School of Osteopathy make regular visits to a residential home for severely disabled individuals in Wandsworth, London, as part of a research study. Under the guidance of tutors, they are currently undertaking an assessment and management plan for four selected residents who are also being regularly assessed by workers at the centre. Changes in these residents are being compared with average figures from the Borough Health Register.

At the Wells Park general practice in Sydenham, South London, an acupuncture and osteopathy service is offered free of charge to patients. The acupuncturist and osteopath work for one day each week, of seven and six hours respectively, in one of the practice's treatment rooms. Between May 1987 and August 1988 the acupuncturist saw 90 patients and the osteopath 107 (Budd *et al.* 1990).

Women can request that an osteopath be with them during labour, if their obstetrician agrees. The osteopath will work on the back, pelvis and diaphragm to relieve pain and to help with breathing.

A group of osteopaths has also been working within the cardio-vascular unit at the Charing Cross Hospital, London (Waldman 1993), which demonstrates that osteopathy has wider uses than simply working on bad backs. The British School of Osteopathy now has a facility and special access for people with a variety of disabilities.

Resources

Training and regulation

In the past there have been five professional organisations repre-senting osteopaths currently practising in the UK: The General Council and Register of Osteopaths, the British and European Osteopathic Association, the Guild of Osteopaths, the College of Osteopaths, and the Natural Therapeutic and Osteopathic Society and Register. All have lists of members which are available to the public. Alternatively, anyone seeking an osteopath can contact the Osteopathic Information Service, which will supply names of local qualified osteopaths.

Osteopathic Information Service
37 Soho Square, London WIV 5DG. *Tel.* 071-439 7177.

When checking the qualifications of an osteopath, the initials after her or his name should include one or other of those in this list:

- MCO   Member of the College of Osteopaths
- DO   Diploma in Osteopathy
- MRO   Member of the Register of Osteopaths
- MLCOM   Member of the London College of Osteopathic Medicine
- MBNOA   Member of the British Naturopathic and Osteopathic Association

In 1993, however, the Osteopaths Bill received Parliamentary assent, and became law. It allows for the setting up in 1995 of a professional body, the General Osteopathic Council, with similar regulations to those governing nurses, doctors and dentists. This governing body will replace the five separate organisations and will set statutory regulations for the registration, training and professional standards of osteopaths. It will also guarantee that all practitioners are covered by professional indemnity insurance.

According to Graham Mason, chairman of the Osteopathic Information Service, 'It will mean patients and GPs who refer them have the security of knowing the osteopath is competent to practise. It also ensures that osteopaths abide by a code of ethics enforceable by law' (*The Times* 1993).

Useful addresses

British and European Osteopathic Association (BEOA)
c/o 15 Station Road, Sidcup, Kent DA15 7EN.

The Association is linked with the Andrew Still College of Osteopathy.

British Naturopathy and Osteopathy Association (BNOA)
6 Netherhall Gardens, London NW3 5RR.

This is the biggest association of naturopaths and osteopaths in Europe. It sets training standards the British College of Naturopathy and Osteopathy (whose site is at the same address) and has a code of ethics for members. Courses are for four years, full-time.

British Osteopathic Association (BOA)
8–10 Boston Place, London NW1 6QH.

The Association is linked to the London College of Osteopathic Medicine, and is for medical doctors only. Courses are for two years, full-time.

College of Osteopaths
110 Thornhill Road, Thames Ditton, Surrey KT7 0UW.

The College was founded in 1948 as a professional organisation for osteopaths. It has a code of ethics and professional conduct. It was one of the eight founder members of the Council for Complementary and Alternative Medicine (see Chapter 1). Courses are for five years, part-time.

General Council and Register of Osteopaths (GCRO)
56 London Street, Reading, Berkshire RG1 4SQ.

The Council, set up in 1936, aims to 'protect the public by insisting on a level of excellence in osteopathic training, practice and behaviour' for members, and governs around three-quarters of all professionally regulated osteopaths in the UK. Membership is open to graduates of schools accredited by the Council.

Guild of Osteopaths (GO)
181 Erith Road, Bexleyheath, Kent DA7 6HS.

Natural Therapeutic and Osteopathic Society and Register (NTOSR)
168 High Street, Maldon, Essex CM9 7BX.

The Society is linked to the London School of Osteopaths. Courses are for five years, part-time.

The College of Osteopaths Practitioners' Association (COPA)
1 Furzehill Road, Borehamwood, Hertfordshire WD6 2DG.

European School of Osteopathy (ESO)
104 Tonbridge Road, Maidstone, Kent ME16 8SL.

Courses are for four years, full-time.

British School of Osteopathy (BSO)
Littlejohn House, 1–4 Suffolk Street, London SWIY 4HG.

Courses are for four years, full-time; various other course structures are under consideration.

Recommended reading

- Belshaw, C. 1987. *Osteopathy – is it for you?* Shaftesbury: Element.
- Littlejohn, J. M. n.d. *The Fundamentals of Osteopathic Technique*. Maidstone: Maidstone Osteopathic Clinic.
- Littlejohn, J. M. n.d. *Principles*. Maidstone: Maidstone College of Osteopathy.
- Master, P. 1988. *Osteopathy for Everyone*. London: Penguin.
- Norminton, T. (ed.) n.d. *A Littlejohn Companion*. Maidstone: Maidstone College of Osteopathy.
- Sandler, S. 1989. *New Ways to Health: a guide to osteopathy*. London: Hamlyn.
- Sandler, S. 1992. *Osteopathy*. London: Macdonald Optima.
- Still, A. T. 1902. *Philosophy of Osteopathy*, reprinted 1977. Colorado Springs, Colorado: American Academy of Osteopathy.
- Stoddard, A. 1980. *The Back: relief from pain*. London: Martin Dunitz.
- Triance, E. 1986. *Osteopathy: a patient's guide*. Wellingborough: Thorson.

Cranial osteopathy

Cranial osteopathy is an extension of osteopathy based on a discovery in the 1930s by an American osteopath, William Garner Sutherland, that the cranial bones that make up the skull are movable and respond to what he termed the **primary respiratory mechanism** (the way in which the intracranial membranes, the brain, the spinal cord and the intra-spinal membranes enclosed within the cerebrospinal fluid fluctuate constantly).

By placing his hand on a client's head, a cranial osteopath can feel the expansion and recession of the cranium and meninges – what practitioners call the **cranial rhythmic impulse** (**CRI**). This is, say practitioners, distinct from the heart rate, respiration and pulse, and there are between 10 and 12 impulses per minute. According to cranial osteopaths, it is possible to pinpoint problems in the body by feeling distortions in the CRI. To correct the distortions a practitioner will gently manipulate the skull and the sacral areas, restoring the balance in the primary respiratory mechanism.

Cranial osteopaths treat a wide range of problems, including headaches, dizziness, fatigue, tinnitus, bronchial congestion, hyperactivity, depression, restlessness, vision problems, conditions arising from congestion (such as the malocclusion of the teeth), and any defect of the senses such as taste or smell. Cranial osteopaths also treat people who have had a head injury – sometimes sorting out problems which the client had not associated with the original accident.

Cranial osteopathy remains largely unknown among health professionals. An exception is Yehudi Gordon, an obstetrician at the Garden Hospital, North London, who recommends that mothers and newborns consult a cranial osteopath if the birth has been arduous. 'Few gynaecologists know about cranial osteopathy or what the technique can do. It's marvellous for the newborn and can iron the stresses and strains of labour. It's important to rule out any underlying pathology in the baby but once that's been excluded, cranial osteopathy is an extremely safe and non-invasive treatment. The effects are superb,' he says (Holmes 1991).

Further reading

- Magoun, H. I. 1976. *Osteopathy in the Cranial Field*. Meridian, Idaho: The Cranial Academy.
- McCatty, R. 1988. *Essentials of Craniosacral Osteopathy*. Bath: Ashgrove Press.
- Sutherland, W. G. 1967. (edited and assembled by Adah Strand Sutherland). *Contributions of Thought*. Produced under the auspices of the Sutherland Cranial Teaching Foundation (no address given).

- Sutherland, W. G. 1948. *The Cranial Bowl: a treatise relating to cranial articular mobility, cranial articular lesions and cranial technique*. Published by the author (now out of print).

The last two of these publications are now very hard to track down, but cranial osteopaths may have copies.

Resources

Cranial osteopathy

Cranial Osteopathic Association
478 Baker Street, Enfield, Middlesex ENI 3QS.

Cranio-Sacral Therapy Education Trust
c/o Karuna Institute, Foxhole, Devon TQ96 6EB.

References

- Budd, C., B. Fisher, D. Parrinder & L. Price 1990. A model of cooperation between complementary and allopathic medicine in a primary care setting. *British Journal of General Practice* **40**: 376–8.
- Campbell, A. 1984. *Natural Health Handbook*. Secaucus, New Jersey; Chartwell Books.
- Consumers Association 1986. Magic or medicine? *Which? Way to Health* (October), 443–7.
- Consumers Association 1993. Osteopathy. *Which? Way To Health* (October), 173–5.
- Giovanna, E. L. & S. Schiowitz 1991. *An Osteopathic Approach to Diagnosis and Treatment*. Philadelphia, Pennsylvania: J. B. Lippincott.
- Holmes, P. 1991. Cranial osteopathy. *Nursing Times* **87**(22): 36–8.
- NAHAT 1993. *Complementary Therapies in the NHS* (Research Paper No. 10). London: National Association of Health Authorities and Trusts.
- Potterton, D. 1978. Osteopathy could herald the end of orthopaedics. *Therapy Weekly* **5**(17): 5.
- Sandler, S. 1992. *Osteopathy*. London: Macdonald Optima.
- Still, A. T. 1897. *Autobiography of A. T. Still*, reprinted 1977. Colorado Springs, Colorado: American Academy of Osteopathy.
- Szmelskyj, A. O., & J. Morris 1992. An investigation of GPs' attitudes to and knowledge of osteopathy. *Complementary Medical Research* **6**(3): 119–23.
- *The Times* 1993. 'Bottom Line': Law to back the osteopath. *The Times*, 26 January.
- Waldman, P. 1993. Osteopathy – an aid to the healing process. *Professional Nurse* **8**(7): 452–4.

16 ALEXANDER TECHNIQUE

Historical background

Unlike most of the techniques and therapies described in this workbook, the history of the Alexander technique is quite recent. Its beginnings can be pinpointed to the late 19th century, to an Australian actor's unpleasant and potentially disastrous experience of losing his voice during performances.

Frederick Matthias Alexander was born in 1869 in North-West Tasmania, the son of a farmer. He survived a rather sickly childhood and left school at sixteen to become a clerk. But his interest in amateur theatricals soon developed into a career, and when he was nineteen he went to Melbourne and became a successful and well-known actor and recitationist.

But as his success increased, he found that his voice became strained and hoarse during performances. On occasion it disappeared completely. Doctors could find no disease or injury to account for the problem, so Alexander decided to find out for himself what was wrong.

He felt that the problem must lie in the way in which he performed, so with the help of mirrors he spent hours watching himself recite, and experimenting to identify what it was about his delivery that caused the loss of voice. An account of this remarkable and ultimately successful exercise in self-study is given in his book, *Use of the Self* (1932).

It was through this painstaking analysis, continued over nearly a decade, that Alexander established the principles of good and bad 'use' of oneself. He overcame his voice problems, and his general health also visibly improved.

Encouraged by his success, he began to teach the technique he had developed for the improvement of use, breathing and voice production. As he developed his teaching skills further, he found that he could more easily convey his ideas if he also used his hands to communicate with his 'pupils' – the method still used today.

Alexander had a thriving teaching practice in Australia and received referrals from doctors. Convinced that his work was of universal value, Alexander was persuaded by the medical profession to take his practice to London in 1904, and he was given letters of recommendation to doctors there.

Once in London, Alexander found enthusiastic supporters among the actors, writers and musicians of the day. George Bernard Shaw, Aldous Huxley, and Henry Irving, for example, all sought his help.

During his life Alexander wrote four books on his technique: *Man's Supreme Inheritance* (1910), *Constructive Conscious Control of the Individual* (1923), *Use of the Self* (1932), and *The Universal Constant in Living* (1942). These books are still in print today (see 'Resources'). In *The Universal Constant in Living* zoologist George Coghill, who was professor at the Wistar Institute of Anatomy and Biology in Philadelphia, wrote an appreciation of Alexander's educational methods; and in *Constructive Conscious Control of the Individual* Professor John Dewey, American educationalist (and brother of the originator of the Dewey decimal system for libraries), wrote the introduction, a critical appraisal of the uniqueness and value of Alexander's educational method.

Alexander travelled to America during the First World War and established the technique there – work that was then continued by his brother. Back in London, in 1931, he set up a training course for teachers of the technique. Alexander continued to work until his death in 1955, after which teachers he had trained went on to offer training to new students. Today there are about five hundred Alexander teachers working throughout the UK.

Further reading

– Westfeldt, L. F. 1964. *Matthias Alexander: the man and his work*. Westport, Connecticut: Associated Booksellers.

What is the Alexander technique?

Next time you travel on public transport, take a look at your fellow travellers. The chances are that they are huddled in corners, or slumped over a paper. It is a sad fact of life that many of us do not use our bodies well. The beautifully poised, upright posture of the young child all too soon transforms into the hunched shoulders and stooped gait of a self-conscious, anxious teenager or weary adult.

Our response to the stresses of life can lead to our skeletal muscles shortening – particularly those associated with the carriage of the head, neck and back. Muscles that have been tightened like this shrink and become locked, and can cause pain and increased tiredness. Poor posture related to slumping or effortful 'holding oneself up' soon becomes a way of life (or 'habit', as Alexander teachers would prefer).

The **Alexander technique** is a method of psycho-physical education by which people learn better use of themselves. The technique operates at a fundamental level – it is about working on our 'use', the ways in which we think and react, and the ways in which we support our bodies and move. Learning the technique allows an individual to become increasingly poised in attitude and movement, and more elastic, fluid and graceful, as potentially self-damaging, awkward, stiff, jerky, and over-hasty and over-tense movements are gradually eliminated.

As the Society of Teachers of the Alexander Technique (see 'Resources') explains:

> posture is far more complex than just standing or sitting up straight. It could be described as how we support and balance our bodies while we go about all our daily activities. From Alexander's own observations, since confirmed by scientific research, it has become apparent that there are natural postural reflexes to organise this support and balance for us without any great effort, provided that we have the necessary understanding and degree of 'relaxation in activity' to allow these to work freely.

Alexander technique practitioners call themselves 'teachers' rather than 'therapists', as they see their role as one of re-education. Clients, in turn, are referred to as 'pupils' or 'students', as their teachers consider they have a collaborative role to play in lessons and are not simply passive recipients of treatment.

An Alexander teacher will show pupils how to release unnecessary tension, and to become more aware of themselves, better aligned and better balanced. According to Kathleen Ballard of the Society of Teachers of the Alexander Technique:

> By words and subtle informed touch pupils are taught how to allow the neck to be free, the head to be released forward and up and the back to lengthen and widen. They learn how to promote this lengthening and freedom when moving from standing to sitting and vice versa. The teacher's touch and advice helps the pupils become aware of habitual misuse and enables them to make changes.

Visiting an Alexander technique teacher

Alexander technique is usually taught on a one-to-one basis in a 30- to 40-minute session, although group lessons can form a useful introduction to the technique. People of any age can benefit from lessons: no one is too old to learn.

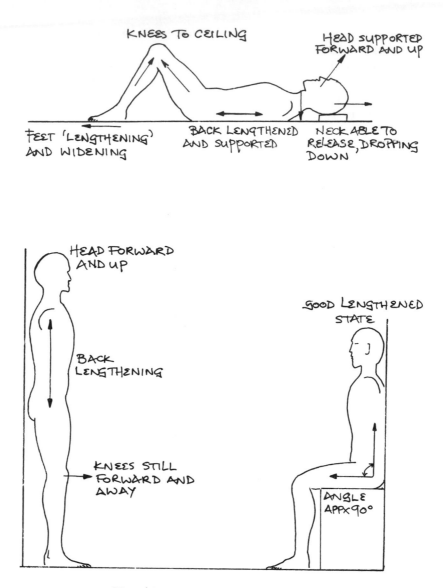

KNEES TO CEILING

HEAD SUPPORTED FORWARD AND UP

FEET 'LENGTHENING' AND WIDENING

BACK LENGTHENED AND SUPPORTED

NECK ABLE TO RELEASE, DROPPING DOWN

HEAD FORWARD AND UP

BACK LENGTHENING

KNEES STILL FORWARD AND AWAY

GOOD LENGTHENED STATE

ANGLE APPX 90°

Fig 16.1: OPTIMUM USE OF THE BODY

Before the lesson starts a pupil is asked to quieten and calm him- or herself, and to bring the attention as fully as possible into the present.

Then the teacher will work with the pupil in a variety of ways. This may involve being asked to sit on a chair. The teacher may touch a pupil's head or back while gently guiding him or her out of and onto the chair. Through this process the pupil will be gradually made aware of poor use of the muscles, and begin learning a new way of sitting, standing and moving (Figure 16.1). Other kinds of movement are explored in lessons, such as crawling, walking, and lifting objects.

Alternatively, a teacher may also work on a student while the student is lying down on a firm surface on his or her back with the knees bent and the head supported by two or three books – this position facilitates the release of over-tight muscles and restores the normal curvature of the spine (Figure 16.1).

In addition to disciplined subtle manual guidance, the teacher will use verbal instructions to help the pupil become aware of the inner **patterns of interference**, and to teach the pupil to project simple messages from the brain to the body that will help the natural mechanisms of poise to function more freely.

Students of the technique have reported sensations of walking on air, of feeling re-energised, and of a greater ease in physical mobility after lessons. Some students also notice physical changes such as the disappearance of a stoop, or the loss of pain in the lower back, neck or shoulder, or the cessation of leg cramps at night. Other benefits may include the ability to stand longer without pain, to walk further without pain and fatigue, to speak and breathe more easily, to think more clearly, and to discipline oneself better. Through learning to acquire poise, the balancing skills improve and fear of falling lessens.

The Alexander technique cannot be learnt overnight, and most teachers would agree that between 20 and 30 lessons will be needed. Initially pupils will usually be asked to attend more than one lesson a week. No special clothing is required, but clothes should not be too bulky or restrict movement.

Further reading

- Gray, J. 1990. *Your Guide to the Alexander Technique*. London: Victor Gollancz.

Indications

Commonly people seek out an Alexander teacher because they have back or neck problems. Others simply want to improve their posture. People who have experienced the technique talk of lasting relief from pain, improvements in physical health and appearance, as well as an increased sense of well-being.

According to the Society of Teachers of the Alexander Technique, the technique can also be helpful for work-related problems such as repetitive strain injuries (now also called 'work-related upper-limb disorder').

People have sought help from the Alexander technique for stress, health promotion, and to prevent problems from occurring.

After undertaking a course of lessons many people find that stress-related conditions, such as migraine or gastro-intestinal conditions are alleviated.

The Alexander technique is popular among musicians and actors for whom poise, grace, ease of speaking and breathing, and economy of movement are essential. Indeed, Alexander technique appears in the curriculum of many acting and music schools, including the Royal Academy of Music and the Royal Academy of Dramatic Art.

Some Alexander teachers go further. Wilfred Barlow, in his book *The Alexander Principle* (1990), suggests that 'the USE is the single most important factor which remains to be dealt with by medical science'. He went on to argue that if this is the case, 'it would be reasonable to expect that its relevance would be most obvious in those medical conditions which, excluding minor coughs and colds, are far and away the greatest cause of general ill-health in our present society'. He believed that in treating any disorder for which physiotherapy is prescribed, the Alexander technique has much to offer. These include rheumatic disorders, spinal disorders, neurological disorders, breathing disorders, antenatal and postnatal care, and rehabilitation.

Dr Barlow, who died in 1991, successfully helped people suffering from epilepsy, claiming a reduction in attacks, and also used the technique to help with a variety of gynaecological conditions, including dysmenorrhoea, retroversion of the uterus, and vaginismus. He concluded, 'The patient feels ill because he has, say, an acute sinus infection, but at the same time he will feel ill because he is using himself badly. The use-patterns which he has developed over the years provide a context which both predisposes him to illness and also diminishes his resilience and capacity to adapt to the stress of the present illness'.

However, to describe the technique as a cure for multifarious forms of malfunction is, in a sense, to trivialise it and mask its true value. It is fundamentally a technique for self-help. Having learnt how to acquire 'good use', however, pupils often find that many health problems related to 'self-misuse' or 'poor use' gradually disappear. These benefits are a 'bonus' – a consequence of learning the technique. Good use goes with mental and physical poise and harmony, the absence of self-damaging conflict of any kind, fluidity of thought, and movement, grace and ease.

Contra-indications

The Alexander technique may not be suitable for people with learning disabilities or people who are mentally disturbed.

Research

Nothing that Alexander has proposed is in conflict with our current understanding of anatomy and physiology. Indeed Nobel physiologist Sir Charles Sherrington acknowledged Alexander's contribution to the physiology of posture and movement, saying that Alexander treated each act as involving the whole integrated individual, with the whole body being involved.

And Professor Raymond Dart, professor of anatomy at Witwatersrand, South Africa, acknowledged receiving helpful instruction from an Alexander teacher which directed his attention to a study of his own postural twists and a theoretical consideration of their origin, in a paper entitled 'Voluntary musculature in the human body – the double spinal arrangement' (Dart 1950).

Early scientific investigation

Scientific investigation of the Alexander technique began after the Second World War, with studies in Britain, for example, by Dr Wilfred Barlow. In his book *The Alexander Technique*, Chris Stevens (1987) details one of Barlow's experiments:

> Barlow gave lessons to a group of 40 students from the Royal College of Music in London. They were photographed in the standard position before and after the course of lessons. Before the course the men had an average of 11 faults and at the end only five. For the women the average faults were reduced from nine to four. These results were compared with a group of 44 students from the Central School of Speech and Drama in London who did not receive Alexander lessons. They were, however, given exercises aimed at improving posture. In this group the men deteriorated slightly from an average of 10.6 faults to 11.7. The women also deteriorated from 7.5 to 7.9.
>
> As a comparison to these two groups, Barlow went on to measure 112 female physical education teacher students. The average number of defects in this group was 8.5.

In the 1950s Professor Frank Pierce-Jones set up experiments at the Institute for Applied Experimental Psychology at Tufts University using multiple-image photography, which demonstrated the effect of the technique on patterns of movement.

– Pierce-Jones, F. 1976. *Body awareness in action: a study of the Alexander technique*. New York: Schocken.

Recent research

Muscle activity

More recent research has recorded muscle activity before, during and after Alexander lessons. Figure 16.2 shows 'a recording from neck muscles which are being trained to release, whilst at the same time, the patient repeats to himself a verbal direction 'neck release'. In (a) there is much initial tension in the neck: in (b) the tension becomes momentarily less, but returns as soon as the teacher stops his gentle adjustment of the head. In (c) the improved balance is obtained sooner, but still it returns when the teacher stops his adjustment and likewise in (d). In (e) the patient is now able to maintain the state of lessened tension and, in time, will be able to evoke this state simply by running over the "orders".'

– Barlow, W. 1990. *The Alexander principle*. London: Victor Gollancz.

Chris Stevens and Professor Finn Boyson-Moller of the University of Copenhagen also used electrical recordings and found that a guided movement required less force and less muscle activity, and was smoother and quicker than the habitual movement.

– Stevens, C. 1987. *The Alexander Technique*. London: Macdonald Optima.

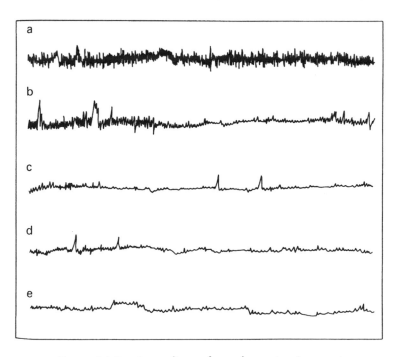

Figure 16.2   *Recordings of muscle tension (see text)*

Respiratory function

In another study John Austin, professor of clinical radiology at the Department of Radiology, Columbia University in New York, investigated the effects of Alexander technique instruction on respiratory function in ten healthy adult volunteers, who each received twenty private Alexander lessons at weekly intervals. Spirometric tests, including maximum static mouth pressures, were assessed before and after each course of lessons. Ten healthy control subjects, matched for age, gender, height and weight, were tested over a similar interval. The group receiving Alexander lessons showed significant increases in peak expiratory flow, maximal voluntary ventilation, and maximal inspiratory mouth pressure. This paper also lists other important research into the Alexander technique.

– Austin, J. H. M. & P. Ausubel 1992. Enhanced respiratory muscular function in normal adults after lessons in proprioceptive musculoskeletal education without exercise. *Chest* 102(2): 486–90.

Chronic back pain

Currently a research investigation of Alexander training in the management of chronic back pain is in progress at Kingston Hospital in London.

Implications for nursing

It takes three years of full-time study to qualify as an Alexander teacher, so the technique is unlikely to be widely incorporated within nursing practice.

However, Alexander teachers Jean Maitland and Harvy Goodliffe (1989) argue that the technique is of value to nurses personally:

> Nearly everybody can benefit from the Alexander technique, but nurses in particular should find it useful, as their working day is extremely demanding. Nurses are constantly on their feet, bending, lifting, carrying and coping with the distress of very sick people. There are often staff shortages, so hours can be long and the pressure constant. Using yourself in a balanced, poised way can help you manage stress. Noticing that you are reacting to a difficult patient by tensing your neck and shoulders will allow you to deal with the stress by freeing the unnecessary tension as it arises.

According to the Society of Teachers of the Alexander Technique, GPs refer patients to Alexander teachers, and some are employing them in health-promotion clinics. A survey of Alexander teachers on low back pain, by the Society (March 1993, unpublished) found that 10 per cent of pupils were referred to them by GPs, and 5 per cent by hospital specialists.

According to STAT, there are also a couple of GPs and nurses who are Alexander technique teachers. Interestingly, according to the National Association of Health Authorities and Trusts (NAHAT 1993), one Family Health Services Authority has given approval to a health-promotion clinic offering Alexander technique.

Nurses, midwives and health visitors should be aware of the benefits of the Alexander technique, and, if it seems that the technique might be appropriate for a patient or client, discuss this option with the client, the doctor and a trained Alexander teacher.

Resources

Training and regulation

Most Alexander teachers are regulated by the Society of Teachers of the Alexander Technique (STAT), and the letters MSTAT after a teacher's name ensures he or she is a member of the Society and will abide by its standards.

The Society was formed in 1958 with these purposes:

- to promote the teaching of the Alexander technique;
- to maintain and improve professional standards;

- to supervise training;
- to prevent exploitation by untrained people;
- to formulate, publish and uphold a code of ethics;
- to deal with infringements;
- to facilitate contact between the public and members;
- to encourage research;
- to organise post-graduate and professional development courses;
- to publish relevant materials.

STAT has codes of professional conduct and ethics, and publishes a regular newsletter and a journal. It is not a member of any of the umbrella organisations that have been set up in the field of complementary medicine. A list of teachers is available if you send an SAE to the Society at the following address:

Society of Teachers of the Alexander Technique (STAT)
London House, 266 Fulham Road, London SW10 9EL.

STAT approves training courses, too, and a list of Alexander teacher training courses is also available from the Society. The standards set were established by Alexander himself and involve three years' full-time training. STAT has a mail-order bookshop, 'Statbooks', which can supply many of the books mentioned in this chapter.

There is also the Alexander Teaching Network which is a professional organisation of Alexander teachers, working mainly in the North, in the North-West and in Scotland. It has a membership of sixty qualified teachers. According to member Jamie McDowell, 'Standards are broadly similar in the two organisations, and involve a full-time three-year training'.

Alexander Teaching Network
PO Box 53, Kendal, Cumbria LA9 4UP.

Recommended reading

- Alexander, F. M. 1910. *Man's Supreme Inheritance*, reprinted 1988. Long Beach, California: Centerline Press.
- Alexander, F. M. 1923. *Constructive Conscious Control of the Individual*, reprinted 1987. London: Victor Gollancz.
- Alexander, F. M. 1932. *Use of the Self*, reprinted 1985. London: Victor Gollancz.
- Alexander, F. M. 1942. *The Universal Constant in Living*, reprinted 1986. Long Beach, California: Centerline Press.
- Barlow, W. 1990. *The Alexander Principle*. London: Victor Gollancz.
- Brennan, R. 1992. *The Alexander Workbook*. Shaftsbury: Element.
- Drake, J. 1991. *Body Know-How*. London: Thorsons.

- Gelb, M. 1987. *Body Learning*. London: Aurum Press.
- Park, G. 1992. *Art of Changing*. Bath: Ashgrove Books.
- Stevens, C. 1991. *Alexander Technique*. London: Optima/Macdonald.

References

- Alexander, F. M. 1910. *Man's Supreme Inheritance*, reprinted 1988. Long Beach, California: Centerline Press.
- Alexander, F. M. 1923. *Constructive Conscious Control of the Individual*, reprinted 1987. London: Victor Gollancz.
- Alexander, F. M. 1932. *Use of the Self*, reprinted 1985. London: Victor Gollancz.
- Alexander, F. M. 1942. *The Universal Constant in Living*, reprinted 1986. Centerline Press.
- Austin, J. H. M. & P. Ausubel 1992. Enhanced respiratory muscular function in normal adults after lessons in proprioceptive musculoskeletal education without exercises. *Chest* **102**(2): 486–90.
- Barlow, W. 1990. *The Alexander Principle*. London: Victor Gollancz.
- Dart, R. 1950. Voluntary musculature in the human body – the double spinal arrangement. *British Journal of Physical Medicine* **13**: 265–8.
- Maitland, J. & H. Goodliffe 1989. The Alexander technique. *Nursing Times* **85**(42): 55–7.
- NAHAT 1993. *Complementary Therapies in the NHS* (Research Paper No. 10). London: National Association of Health Authorities and Trusts.
- Pierce-Jones, F. 1976. *Body Awareness in Action: a study of the Alexander technique*. New York: Schocken.
- Stevens, C. 1987. *The Alexander Technique*. London: Macdonald Optima.

17 RESEARCH

There are many vexed issues in complementary therapies, but none arouses as much sound and fury as the question of **research**.

This is surprising, for every time a therapist treats someone, he or she is experimenting with subtle differences in technique, noting what works and what doesn't and building up a store of knowledge: this is a form of research in itself. If one discusses the subject with practitioners for a while, though, it soon becomes clear that in most cases where there is a strongly-held feeling on the subject, the real issue is **validation**, not research *per se*.

There are several schools of thought among therapists, it seems. The first of these is 'I know that therapy X works, because I have seen and/or experienced for myself the benefits it brings.' People holding this belief deem research unnecessary, because it would only tell them what they know already: it would be like running a clinical trial to establish whether or not aspirin brings down high temperatures.

Next is 'Holistic therapies cannot be subjected to the "scientific" method of setting up a hypothesis and then trying to disprove it, because there are too many variables involved: every patient is unique.' For this group, accepted research methods are not powerful enough to generate meaningful data, and so can be dispensed with in favour of case study meta-analysis (see Box 17.1).

A more complex argument, which relates mainly to therapies with roots in non-Western philosophy or medicine, is this: 'Normal research methods, applied to therapy Y, fall down if the underlying principles are not accepted.' Thus if the given therapy postulates a 'vital force', for example, Western scientific method is of little use if the findings have to be interpreted in terms of Western science, which does not recognise the existence of that particular form of energy.

The final objection, which comes in two forms, both extremely difficult to counter, takes this form: 'If the scientific method is unable to show how therapy Z works, all that demonstrates is that science is not yet advanced enough to do so; we need a paradigm shift' (Laffan 1993).

During the course of this book's preparation, all these arguments have been put to us by practitioners, sometimes apologetically, sometimes defiantly, when we have asked about the lack of published research in some therapies. Before going any further, perhaps we should stop and ask the implicit question: why should any therapy have to be validated at all?

Orthodox Western medicine, it should be made clear, cannot claim to be a completely scientifically-tested discipline: it has been estimated that only 15 per cent of practice is based on 'sound science' (Eddy & Billings 1993). The idea that medical doctors base all their practice on rigorously-tested theory is simply untrue: it is as false as the idea that all complementary medical practitioners eschew research-based practice. Texts of medical ethics, where real-life case studies are presented for discussion, highlight how much of orthodox practice is based on what can only be described as 'intuition', the sifting and weighing of evidence below the level of consciousness, to arrive at a plan of action that is 'correct' (Ackerman & Strong 1989).

On the whole, though, among practitioners of complementary medicine, it is taken for granted that research-based practice is essential for delivery a high standard of care within the field: 'research into complementary therapies is urgently needed' (Bell 1987), and the work must be of an acceptable quality' (Tonkin 1987), according to just two experts. Without such study, dogma can take precedence over enquiry, with the result that improvements may never be made, and less effective practices may be perpetuated. The Research Council for Complementary Medicine has spent more than a decade in persuading practitioners of the importance of research validation, giving help when and where possible, and the increasingly high quality of published work is a testimony to their efforts; but there is still some way to go, possibly because some practitioners do not have a clear understanding of what 'research' entails.

All clinical trials seek to *disprove* a hypothesis; if they fail to do so, then the reliability of the hypothesis is seen as being that much stronger. Attempting to *prove* something is likely to result in alternative, possibly correct, hypotheses not being considered.

A weakness in some complementary medical research is that the authors fail to acknowledge this principle, and this is probably the commonest reason why *Nursing Times*, to name the journal with which we ourselves are most familiar, rejects some submitted studies. If a researcher looks at the use of a particular therapy, and starts from the position that 'This achieves these results because ...', the study is doomed from the start.

Consider this example: I have a theory that tea is a powerful therapeutic tool, and set out to prove it. Firstly, I look at patients on a hospital ward, and look at what happens when they engage in tea-drinking behaviour. Anyone drinking anything else is of course excluded from the study, as they are irrelevant.

In study period 1, at breakfast time, I notice that a stuporous state is quickly lifted when people drink tea. This tells me that tea is a powerful stimulant, operating directly on the nervous system, raising neutrological function over time.

In study period 2, mid-morning, I go down to the dayroom and note that tea drinkers are talking together. Again, this suggests that we are dealing with a neurologically effective agent, acting directly to improve psychological status.

During study period 3, at lunchtime, I note the recurrence of this effect, but note that many of the tea drinkers express a wish to have a nap afterwards. This proves the neuostimulant effect, because these patients have obviously been overstimulated, with a concomitant protective rest mechanism coming into action.

And so on … If I had tried to *disprove* the hypothesis, and so sought *other* reasons to explain the effects I noted, the outcome of my 'research' would have been very different, and a lot more informative.

This may seem an extreme example, and it is not intended to be taken seriously; nevertheless, there have been worse experimental designs in actual research work which practitioners have later sought to publish.

BOX 17.1
SOME RESEARCH TERMINOLOGY

Experimental design is intended to minimise the effects of chance. The following techniques are part of this process.

Randomisation

All subjects in a trial should have an equal chance of being in any groups that exist, and so must be *individually* randomised. Imagine a study looking at staff punctuality in a ward, and factors affecting it; and suppose further that it was necessary to consider the staff in two groups: the results could be seriously damaged by putting the first three people to arrive on duty into one group, and the next three into the other, although superficially this appears to be 'randomisation'.

Control

To establish whether or not a given intervention is the *reason* for an observed difference, there must be a control group with which to compare the study group. This group is treated identically to the study group, with the single exception that members do not receive the intervention. Consider, for example, a study of whether digestive biscuits produce an elevation in mood mid-morning: this would have a study group receiving biscuits, while the controls would be given something of equal calorific value. If a difference between groups were observed, possible explanations like 'raised blood-glucose levels' could probably be ruled out, clearing the field for further investigation.

Placebo

A placebo is an inert substance or a non-effective treatment, but the person receiving it does not know this. The most obvious example is in drug trials: all subjects receive a plain pill or capsule, but only the study group get the active substance.

Placebo control is important in research, because the very act of being treated, even when the treatment itself is ineffective, can produce some kind of result. Oddly enough, though, one study showed that even if patients were told they were being given a placebo, there were still therapeutic effects from it (Park & Covi 1965).

Saying 'it's just the placebo effect' is one of the most intellectually lazy arguments used by opponents of complementary therapy. The placebo effect is a powerful therapeutic tool, whose use is little understood; if measurable changes in health are effected, for whatever reason, it cannot simply be written off as 'placebo' just because the researcher cannot identify any simpler cause.

Blinding

The 'blinding' procedure involves some of the people involved in a trial not knowing whether placebo or active treatment is being given – usually members of the study group. In a double-blind trial, the people giving the treatment do not know which is which, either; this is to avoid any subtle differences between the way they deal with subjects and controls caused by their knowledge and picked up by the recipients of the treatment at a level below consciousness. If this is impossible – for example, in a study of massage – then it is the *assessors* of any effects who are 'blinded'. Blinding is removed only after the trial has run its course, and individual responses have been analysed and tabulated.

Crossover

In a crossover trial, groups receive one treatment for a period of time, and then another. In our digestive biscuit study, for example, half the subjects might receive biscuits in the first week and calorific equivalents in the second, while in the other group this order would be reversed.

Prospective and retrospective studies

In a prospective study, the subjects are identified and randomised beforehand. For example, research into patients' falls from bed might take all patients coming onto one ward in a month, and chart their progress, with half having cot sides on their beds and half not, completely at random. A retrospective study might look at all patients who fell in the ward over a month, and draw conclusions from whether or not they had had cot sides on their beds.

Statistical significance

A finding is said to be significant if statistically there is only a very small probability of the given result being achieved by chance. The greatest accepted significance level is 5 per cent – a 1 in 20 probability of it being a *chance* result. Related to this, there are many well-tried statistical techniques that enable a researcher to establish the *minimum number* of subjects required if the study is to be of value.

Meta-analysis

If individual studies are deemed to be too small for meaningful conclusions to be drawn, it is sometimes legitimate to group together a number of similar studies and to analyse their findings collectively. This is a very useful technique, but can produce unreliable and perhaps misleading results if the choice of studies for inclusion is not conducted scrupulously.

There are many other types of trial, but these are techniques of which examples can be found in the research sections of individual chapters within this book.

Further reading

- Bailer, J. C. & F. Mosteller (eds) 1992. *Medical Uses of Statistics*, 2nd edn. Boston, Massachusetts: NEJM Books.
- Darling, V. H. & J. Rogers 1986. *Research for Practising Nurses*. London: Macmillan.
- Huff, D. 1954. *How To Lie with Statistics*, reprinted 1973. Harmondsworth: Penguin.

Anecdotal evidence

There is nothing 'unscientific' about **anecdotal evidence**, it seems, provided it is identifiable as such. It may be called a **case report,** a **case study** (Liebrich 1990), or – if the researcher has sufficient professional status – **personal observations**. The value of case studies is well recognised; much of the literature in neurology would have to be dispensed with, if such reports were ruled out of use.

Criticisms of anecdotal evidence in complementary therapies appear to centre around the lack of background information. If a psychiatrist, for example, has published in the *British Journal of Psychiatry* a report of a particularly unusual pattern of behaviour in a client, and how he or she dealt with it, the readers are likely to have some experience of clients with similar, if not identical, behaviour; they can compare the author's conclusions with their own, based on this background experiential knowledge. If the therapy is one that is unfamiliar to its audience that grounding may be lacking: all that the reader, unversed in the therapy, can do is accept or reject the author's conclusions as he or she thinks fit.

Where case studies could come into their own is if they were seen for what they are: foundation stones, and not the building itself. Reading a number of studies helps the reader to get a 'feel' for the therapy, but further information is still needed: are these cases 'typical' in any way, enabling trends and common features to be identified? Is the author only presenting successes – how many people has he or she treated in this way, and were any outcomes similar or different? Were the treatments the same, or did they vary at all? What significance does this hold?

Uncontrollable variables

Even a quick comparison of the leading medical journals of today, and ten years ago, will show how **statistics** have come to the fore. This may be something to do with easier access to powerful computing equipment, and systems designed purely for use in health-care research; the principles remain the same, however.

The value of the sophisticated statistical tools currently available is that the effects of chance can be scrutinised more closely. This weakens the argument about individual response differences negating the possibility of research – but only if the **sample** sizes used are sufficiently large.

It is a potential weakness of orthodox medical research, not often recognised, that patient individuality is not always given the attention it deserves: 'All too often, in our concern to demonstrate whether or not one therapy is better/safer/cheaper/more comfortable/less dangerous than another, we fall into the trap of deceiving ourselves that our treatment is in itself the only factor to be taken into account, and that the patient's individuality is irrelevant to the healing process. The truth is that variation in the patient's response to a particular remedy or therapeutic activity is a key element in determining the degree of benefit (or detriment) that any individual patient may derive from any particular treatment – orthodox or complementary' (Tonkin 1987). This suggestions that a synthesis of conventional and non-conventional practitioners' views on this aspect of research could be of benefit to all concerned.

Accepting the underlying principles

When a complementary practitioner asks readers of his or her research to take some things on trust, either implicitly or explicitly, alarm bells should start ringing. Without some kind of discussion about the reasons *why* the author believes the underlying theory to be sound, everything that follows is hard to accept.

Reflexology (Chapter 5) provides an example of this. The idea that different areas of the body are 'reflected' onto areas of the skin is not a completely unsubstantiated assertion; neurological studies of the 19th century first suggested that this may be the case, and as we saw in the chapter, 'referred pain' is a well-known phenomenon. But when practitioners produce diagrams that say 'Here is the gallbladder reflex', there should be some kind of evidence of that connection. Honest practitioners say, 'I *believe* the connection exists, because my experience with patients has led me to believe that it is so; the underlying mechanism might be related to embryonic co-development of nerve supplies, stimulation of the lymphatic system, removal of lactic-acid residues, or some as yet unknown mechanism, but I don't know for sure.' But there are others who imply, 'This is so, and needs no further evidence', when they produce work that fails to address possible mechanisms involved. It is interesting that of all the therapies discussed in this book, reflexology is the only one for which we were unable to find a single piece of published evidence for its postulated mechanism of action. This is not to say that reflexology is worthless – there are too many people who have derived benefit from the treatment for such an assertion to be made – but its full potential is wasted, if avenues for research are closed off by dogmatism.

Traditional Chinese medicine (TCM) seems to raise the same problems. There is no evidence for the existence of Qi, and its routes around the body are unsupported by current neurological theory, some texts relying on repetition of the (unreferenced) story of a man hit by lightning, who apparently described new sensory pathways that corresponded to the classic descriptions of the Meridians. Yet TCM has been subjected to such an amount of testing, both qualitative and quantitative, that pratitioners have earned the right to say, 'This may not fit in with your received knowledge, but the system constitutes a self-contained and consistent whole, with proven outcomes.' Research into TCM, like the studies on herbal treatments for childhood eczema (Sheehan & Atherton 1992), stand out as being methodologically sound, even when looked at in terms of Western scientific method, because 'TCM satisfies the following scientific criteria: it is based on observation over a long period of time; it has been tried, tested and refined; it has its own coherent and self-consistent theoretical

framework; its effects are predictable within its own framework'
(McGourty 1993).

If a practitioner says that research is impossible without a leap of
faith, then it is hard not to question the validity of the underlying
theory.

The shortcomings of science and 'the needed paradigm shift'

This is a very hard argument to counter, but to dismiss a therapy
completely, saying it is 'unscientific', is in itself unscientific, as well
as intellectually lazy (see Box 17.2).

Naturopathy (Chapter 12) was called unscientific and a crank
medicine for a long time, but its principle of 'let nature be the
healer' and its advocacy of fresh food, water and air are now parts
of orthodox medicine. Its early practitioners said that science had
to catch up with them and they were proved right.

A therapy on the cusp is Therapeutic Touch (Chapter 7). This
appears to have moved away from its early Eastern philosophical
base, and connections with healing by 'laying on of hands',
towards integration with quantum physics and a belief that the
entire universe is a single energy field, with life being a part of it.
Whether proponents of this theory are right or wrong will not be
known for some time, in all probability; but again, these ideas
cannot be dismisssed out of hand.

However, it is too easy for anyone to say, 'If you don't understand what I am doing, that's a pointer to *your* ignorance, not mine'.
The theory underlying any therapy must be tested in the light of
current knowledge; if it does not fit, that does not necessarily mean
that current knowledge is wrong. Only after rigorous intellectual
enquiry has been carried out should anyone start talking about
paradigm shifts (jargon for 'a new way of looking at things').

BOX 17.2
**SCIENTIFIC SCEPTICISM AND COMPLEMENTARY MEDICAL
RESEARCH**

Writing in the *Nursing Times* 'Arena' column in 1988, Colin Brewer,
medical director of the Stapleford Addiction Centre, London, said:
'Hardly a day goes by without some new "therapy" being touted as
providing not merely relief, but a lasting cure for conditions as diverse
as cancer, depression and eczema. What virtually all "alternative"

treatments have in common is that they have never been subjected to anything that could be described as a controlled trial (Brewer 1988).

As the research sections for almost all the therapies in this book have shown, this is patently untrue, but Dr Brewer's view is still a common one. The fact is that there are many people who continue to claim that complementary therapy remains 'unproven', regardless of any evidence to the contrary. Worse still, there are those who actively seek to discredit the whole field – sometimes in ways that can only be described as underhand.

The notorious study investigating the Bristol Cancer Help Centre (BCHC) is a case in point. The interim report, published in 1990 (Bagenal et al. 1990), suggested that women with breast cancer who supplemented conventional treatment with the régime advocated by the BCHC were twice as likely to relapse as women treated with 'conventional' methods. The media trumpeted these 'results' on the front pages of newspapers, and as lead stories on television and radio news bulletins, and groups and individuals opposed to the use of complementary therapies had a field day.

The subsequent letter of retraction, which acknowledged that 'the difference could be explained by increasing severity of disease in BCHC attenders' (Chilvers et al. 1990), did not receive nearly so much attention, and several years later the centre is still trying to repair the damage done (Weir 1993).

When research is published that appears, in any way, to add weight to claims for the effectiveness of complementary therapies, the opposition's voices can usually be heard crying 'fluke' or 'it's just the placebo effect'. If these objections do not have the required effect, there may be more damaging accusations levelled against the researchers.

A French research team found that an aqueous solution of an anti-body retained its ability to evoke a biological response, even when diluted past the point where the likelihood of even a single molecule of the original substance being left was negligible. The leading science journal, Nature, published the results (Davenas et al. 1988), then sent its editor, a magician (to 'test for trickery') and an expert in the field of scientific misconduct to investigate.

The study was not intended to be a 'proof' of homoeopathy (Chapter 10), but it certainly lent weight to the therapy's most widely debated principle, concerning potency and dilution. Yet it seemed to worry the Nature team: despite the fact that five other laboratories had replicated the findings prior to the study's publication, the journal's representatives concluded after their visit that 'the [French] laboratory has fostered, and then cherished, a delusion about the interpretation of its data' (Maddox et al. 1988). The magician, James Randi, went on to say specifically that the results were a 'fraud'.

Professor Beneviste, head of the research team, should be complimented on his restraint after such behaviour, and many will applaud his response: 'Salem witch hunts or McCarthy-like prosecutions will kill science ... The only way definitively to establish conflicting results is to reproduce them. It may be that all of us are wrong in good faith. This is no crime, but science as usual, and only the future knows' (Beneviste 1988).

It is the light shed by subsequent studies of the work of Beneviste's team that will move 'science' forward; the unsubstantiated cries of 'fraud' simply put the scientific process of open inquiry into reverse.

It seems that few opportunities to highlight the failures of complementary medicine are missed. For example, a young man called Grant Grove rejected orthodox treatment for Hodgkin's disease in favour of a cocktail of complementary therapies, and died two years later; the television programme in which his case was discussed (*Public Eye*, BBC2, 29 January 1993) and subsequent newspaper report (*Today* 1993) used his death as a warning against the use of complementary therapies. Very few people, especially health-care professionals, do not know of someone who died while receiving 'orthodox' medical treatment, but how many would take an individual example and hold it up as 'proof' that such medicine was ineffective, and should be banned forthwith?

Conclusion

The weight of evidence for some complementary therapies' efficacy is building up, but as long as individual practitioners continue to claim that their particular speciality should be exempt from scrutiny, then sceptics will remain unconvinced, and health-care professionals wanting to know more will be deterred from making the effort. The work of researchers in attempting to prove or disprove hypotheses about therapies is moving the limits of knowledge outwards, but it takes a lot of trials to counterbalance just one zealot's words, when these are quoted widely and disparagingly by individuals and groups who are, for whatever reason, opposed to the integration of complementary medicine into the mainstream.

A paper was submitted to *Nursing Times*, sometime ago, by a medical practitioner concerned about the use of a particular therapy in his hospital by nurses who could offer little in the way of rationale for their treatments; his literature search turned up some statements by 'researchers' that made it easy to pour scorn on that therapy, being full of words and phrases like 'obviously', 'which therefore proves', and other *non sequiturs*. (It was suggested that he might like to look at some more balanced and rational papers on the subject, before re-submitting his own).

This is just one example of something for which (admittedly anecdotal) evidence is mounting: the rejection of the need of research is harming the chance of potentially beneficial therapies being properly investigated.

Yet as we have seen, the prospective, double-blind, randomised, placebo-controlled crossover trial is not the only way of conducting a study into complementary therapies. What is needed is honest enquiry: catalogue the successes by all means, but let the failures be recorded, too. In the short term, this may provide ammunition for people whose minds are closed to the potential of some therapies; but in the long term, it is the only way that potential will be realised.

References

- Ackerman, T. F. & C. Strong 1989. *A Casebook of Medical Ethics*. Oxford: Oxford University Press.
- Bagenal, F. S., D. F. Easton, E. Harris, *et al.* 1990. Survival of patients with breast cancer attending Bristol Cancer Help Centre. *Lancet* **336** (8715): 606–10.
- Bell, C. M. J. 1987. How can individual practitioners contribute to research? *Complementary Medical Research* **2**(2): 168–74.
- Beneviste, J. 1988. Beneviste on the Beneviste affair. *Nature* **335**: 759.
- Brewer, C. 1988. No alternative. *Nursing Times* **84**(41): 24.
- Chilvers, C. E. D., D. F. Easton, F. S. Bagenal, *et al.* 1990. Bristol Cancer Help Centre (letter). *Lancet* **336**(8724): 1189–90.
- Davenas, E., F. Beauvais, J. Amara, *et al.* 1988. Human basophil degranulation triggered by very dilute antiserum against IgE. *Nature*. **333**: 816–18.
- Eddy, D. M. & J. D. Billings 1993. The quality of medical evidence and medical practice. Paper prepared for the National Leadership Commission on Health Care. Cited in Buckman, R. & K. Sabbagh 1993: *Magic or Medicine? An investigation into healing*. London: Macmillan.
- Laffan, G. 1993. A new holistic science. *Nursing Standard* **7**(17): 44–5.
- Liebrich, J. 1990. Measurement of efficacy: a case for holistic research. *Complementary Medical Research*. **4**(1): 21–5.
- Maddox, J., J. Randi & W. W. Stewart 1988. 'High-dilution' experiments a delusion. *Nature* **334**: 291.
- McGourty, H. 1993. *How to Evaluate Complementary Therapies: a literature review*. (Observatory Report Series: 13) Liverpool: Liverpool Public Health Observatory.
- Park, L. C. & L. Covi 1965. Nonblind placebo trial. *Archives of General Psychiatry* **12**: 336–45. Cited in Buckmann, R. & K. Sabbagh 1993: *Magic or Medicine? An investigation into healing*. London: Macmillan, Chapter 8 – this has a detailed discussion of the placebo effect.
- Sheehan, M. P. & D. J. Atherton 1992. A controlled trial of traditional Chinese medicinal plants in widespread non-exudative eczema. *British Journal of Dermatology* **126**:179–84.

- *Today* 1993. Let the myth of natural medicine die here with me. *Today,* 29 January.
- Tonkin, R. 1987. Research into complementary medicine. *Complementary Medical Research* **2**(1): 3–9.
- Weir, M. W. 1993. Bristol Cancer Help Centre: successes and setbacks, but the journey continues. *Complementary Therapies in Medicine* **1**(1) 42–5.

BOX 17.3
COMPLEMENTARY MEDICINE INDEX

Complementary Medicine Index is one of four monthly titles derived from AMED, the bibliographic database produced by the Medical Information Centre. Each issue contains citations organised into broad subject categories and indexes to authors and subjects. Most months contains around 300 citations, and annual cumulations of the individual indexes are available. The database currently contain more than 60 000 records from 1985 and is growing at about 800 records per month. The literature of complementary medicine, including major areas like acupuncture, homoeopathy and herbalism and a range of allied health topics (physiotherapy, occupational therapy and rehabilitation) is covered comprehensively from journals collected by the British Library Document Supply Centre. Most journal parts are processed within two weeks of their arrival.

The database is also available online, through Datastar and MIC-KIBIC (Stockholm, Sweden), and on floppy discs as subsets of the records, corresponding to the main topics of the database. These can be supplied together with Idealist database software, ready for loading into personal computers. Also available are individual searches processed by staff of the Medical Information Centre.

Further information, including prices, can be obtained from:

Medicine Information Centre, British Library DSC
Boston Spa, Wetherby, West Yorkshire LS23 7BQ. *Tel.* 0937 546039; *fax* 0937 546458.

18 CONCLUSION

It is clear that there are many encouraging initiatives currently taking place in the field of non-conventional therapy, and it is hoped that good practice in each can be extrapolated for general use.

A quote from a supportive commentator, a therapist, or perhaps a satisfied client? In fact it is just one of the conclusions the British Medical Association came to in its recent investigation of complementary medicine (BMA 1993). If the gamekeeper has now turned poacher, surely complementary medicine has come of age?

The very fact that we have written this book attests to how far complementary medicine has come. In it we have documented the rise in consumer interest, the increased professionalism of therapists, the accumulation of useful research, and lastly what appear to be the beginnings of the integration of complementary medicine within the health service.

Nursing's interest in complementary medicine is relatively recent, and has been fuelled in part by a desire by many nurses to get back to the bedside and the patient – to provide hands-on caring (see Chapter 2). A small (unpublished) survey conducted by *Nursing Times* in 1993 found that an astonishing 92 per cent of nurses, midwives and health visitors who responded were interested in complementary therapies and in training in this area, 88 per cent would like to use complementary therapies in the future, and 78 per cent said that they either used complementary therapies, or recommended their use to patients. We believe it important that this enthusiasm be tempered by a firm understanding of the therapies concerned and the limitations to their use: from this belief the idea for a comprehensive book for nurses, midwives and health visitors was born.

That only 14 of the 160 or so therapies known to exist have been included in this book was a deliberate decision. We selected therapies that we felt would be of interest to a large number of nurses, midwives and health visitors, and that had reasonably good training standards and regulations for practitioners. In subsequent editions our list may well expand to include more therapies, as these become better known and better established.

The question must now be whether the integration of complementary medicine within nursing, and within the health service generally, is a permanent change or a 'passing fad'. And if the integration is permanent, is it actually a good thing?

Let us take nursing first. The changes that have swept through education, practice and management in recent years have turned nurses into far more autonomous and professional practitioners, practitioners who are better equipped to develop their profession along the lines they believe appropriate. Many nurses see in complementary therapies ideal skills for nurses to acquire in order to extend their practice. With ward sisters and charge nurses becoming budget holders, for example, the incorporation of complementary therapies into the care offered by nurses on a particular ward becomes a much more straightforward proposition. If done well, this can only be good for the patient, although – as we pointed out in Chapter 2 – it may not always be the best use of resources to train nurses in complementary therapies in preference to 'buying in' the services of professional complementary therapists.

A potential problem with the use of complementary medicine by nurses is the current lack of evaluation. Without evaluation of the therapeutic value of a particular therapy it will be difficult for nurses to justify its use – or the resources it requires. This alone may prevent the widespread use of therapies that might well have a variety of therapeutic benefits for patients.

It is also true that it would not reflect well on the profession if untested, and unevaluated, therapies were being used in the care of very sick people.

At the moment complementary therapies are enjoying enormous popularity among nurses, but there is a possibility that this will not last. Complementary medicine has had other phases of general popularity – the 1930s being the last – after which they have sunk again into obscurity. If this is not to happen within nursing, the profession must ensure that nurses receive appropriate training, conduct good-quality research, and find ways of formally incorporating the use of complementary therapies within their practice.

And what about the health service as a whole? Certainly there appears to be the political will to allow the integration of complementary therapies into the health service (see Chapter 1), and in the event of a Labour government coming to power, that party certainly appears keen to continue the trend. Moreover, the National Association of Health Authorities and Trusts found in its survey of purchasers that there is a willingness to pay for complementary therapies for patients (NAHAT 1993). A lack of funding for health care is likely to limit the availability of such services, however.

Making complementary therapies available on the NHS will allow more people to use them. Many would like to use them now, but cannot afford the fees that therapists must charge if they are to make a living.

However, bringing complementary therapies into the NHS raises important issues relating to the therapies themselves – which therapies should be available on the NHS, how the competence of therapists will be assessed, how the effectiveness of the therapy itself will be assessed, and so on. Currently, the use of complementary therapies within the NHS has been somewhat ad hoc, with little co-ordination and few agreed methods of evaluation.

We only need a few deaths attributed to complementary medicine for the whole process to be reversed. As the BMA suggests, what is needed is 'that each body representing a therapy demonstrate: an organized structure; a single register of members; guidelines on relationships with medical practitioners; sound training at accredited institutions; an effective ethical code; agreed levels of competence; and a proven commitment to research. Such features not only safeguard the patient from possible harm, but also provide practitioners of the therapy with a recognized status' (BMA 1993).

We believe – and we hope this book demonstrates it – that complementary medicine does have an important role to play in health care. We believe that nurses should have the opportunity – should they so wish – to incorporate particular therapies within their practice. We know this is what patients want. What we now hope is that nurses, midwives and health visitors, along with other health professionals in the health service, will work together with complementary therapists to ensure that this happens in a thorough and effective manner.

References

- BMA 1993. *Complementary Medicine: new approaches to good practice.* London: British Medical Association.
- NAHAT 1993. *Complementary therapies in the NHS* (Research Paper No. 10). London: National Association of Health Authorities and Trusts.

INDEX

rheumatoid arthritis 81, 125, 161
rhinitis 175
Rogers, Martha 88, 89
Rose 75
Rosemary 75
Royal College of Nursing
  Institute of Advanced Nursing Education 36, 40
  special interest group in complementary medicine 11, 23, 87
  training in complementary therapies 15

sampling 232
Sandalwood 75
Sassafras bark 148, 149
Sayre-Adams, Jean 88, 90–1
School of Herbal Medicine 154
Schuessler, Wilhelm 118, 135
sciatica 31, 175, 207
science 234–6
  and validation 227–8
Scottish College of Homoeopathy 134
scurvy 102
self-help 5
  Alexander technique 223–4
  herbal medicine 148
  homoeopathy 123–5
  massage 32
self-hypnosis 113, 114
sexual problems 112, 176, 220
Shen 167
shiatsu 43–55
  definition and theory 44–7
  history 43
  indications and contra-indications 50–1
  and nursing 53
  research 51–2
  training and regulation 54
  treatment 47–50
Shiatsu Society 54
significance, statistical 231
simples 144
sinusitis 175
skin oils and lotions 71–2
skin problems 31, 63, 76, 112, 122, 176, 186
skull, osteopathy 212–13
smoking, giving up 181
Society of Homoeopaths 121, 122, 132

Society for the Promotion of Nutritional Therapy 100
Society of Teachers of the Alexander Technique 217, 219, 224–5
spine 205
  and Alexander technique 218
  and central nervous system 192
  and chiropractic 191–3
  and osteopathy 200, 204, 208
sports, and complementary therapies 31, 207
Staphysagria 124
statistics 231, 232
Still, Andrew Taylor 200, 201–2
stress
  and Alexander technique 216, 219–20
  and aromatherapy 76, 80
  and homoeopathy 124
  and hypnotherapy 112
  and massage 30, 35, 37
  and reflexology 63, 64
  and shiatsu 50
  and Therapeutic Touch 92
succussion 119
suggestion 110, 111
surveys 5, 6–8
  Consumers' Association 7–8, 207
  Daily Telegraph 6–7, 10–11
  homoeopathy 128
  Medical Care Research Unit 7
  NAHAT (*q.v.*) 9–10, 20, 240
  Nursing Times 239
  osteopathy 207
  Taylor Nelson Medical 5
  Threshold Foundation 5
Sussex School of Massage 41
Sutherland, William Garner 201, 210
Swedish massage 26, 30

tanden 45
Tao 167, 185
Tao-Yinn 43
tapotement 27–8, 29
Tea tree 75
tenosynovitis 207
terminal patients 38
thalamic pain 51
therapeutic relationship 110
Therapeutic Touch (TT) 88–95
  definition and theory 89–90, 233